DIGESTIVE DISEASES - RESEARCH AND CLINICAL DEVELOPMENTS

SHORT BOWEL SYNDROME IN CHILDREN

CURRENT PRACTICE AND FUTURE PERSPECTIVES

DIGESTIVE DISEASES – RESEARCH AND CLINICAL DEVELOPMENTS

Additional books in this series can be found on Nova's website under the Series tab.

Additional e-books in this series can be found on Nova's website under the e-book tab.

DIGESTIVE DISEASES - RESEARCH AND CLINICAL DEVELOPMENTS

SHORT BOWEL SYNDROME IN CHILDREN

CURRENT PRACTICE AND FUTURE PERSPECTIVES

IGOR SUKHOTNIK, M.D.
EDITOR

NOVA BIOMEDICAL

New York

For permission to use material from this book please contact us:
Telephone 631-231-7269; Fax 631-231-8175
Web Site: http://www.novapublishers.com

Library of Congress Cataloging-in-Publication Data

ISBN: 978-1-62948-518-8

Published by Nova Science Publishers, Inc. † New York

Contents

In: Short Bowel Syndrome in Children
Editor: Igor Sukhotnik
ISBN: 978-1-62948-518-8

Chapter I

Short Bowel Syndrome: Definition, Incidence, Historical Overview and Etiology

I. Sukhotnik, M.D.
Department of Pediatric Surgery, Bnai Zion Medical Center,
Technion-Israel Institute of Technology,
The Ruth & Bruce Rappaport Faculty of Medicine, Haifa, Israel

Abstract

Short bowel syndrome (SBS) is defined as a condition of malabsorption that is due to reduction of functional intestinal mass necessary for adequate digestion and absorption for nutrient, fluid and growth requirements. SBS typically follows resection of 50% or more of the small intestine and is associated with diarrhea, steatorrhea, dehydration, electrolyte disturbances, malabsorption and progressive malnutrition. SBS is a functional rather than anatomic entity and its definition may be based on the need for intervention: patients requiring parenteral nutrition support for more than 1 to 3 months after massive small bowel resection can be defined as having SBS. The incidence of TPN-dependent SBS patients is estimated between 2 and 3 per million per year, with the prevalence at approximately 4 per year per million. In pediatric populations, SBS occurs in newborns and infants suffering from necrotizing enterocolitis, intestinal atresias, long-segment Hirschsprung's disease and malrotation with volvulus requiring massive intestinal resection. In adults, extensive resection is related to mesenteric vascular accidents, malignancy, radiation strictures, adhesive obstruction and Crohn's disease. Other etiologies include trauma, fistula, scleroderma, radiation enteritis and intestinal obstruction. SBS has significant morbidity and is potentially lethal especially when intestinal loss is extensive.

Keywords: Short bowel syndrome, intestinal failure, bowel resection, children, infants, adult, definition, intestinal length, functional capability, total parenteral nutrition, historical overview, etiology, incidence

A. Definition of Short Bowel Syndrome

Short bowel syndrome (SBS) can be defined as the critical loss of intestinal length or competence below the minimal amount necessary for the adequate digestion and absorption to satisfy body nutrient and fluid requirements for maintenance in normal nutritional status in adults or promote appropriate growth in children [1-3]. SBS is associated with diarrhea, steatorrhea, electrolyte disturbances, dehydration, malabsorption and progressive malnutrition requiring parenteral nutrition (PN) as long as it persists.

Definition of SBS remains a matter of debate. Many investigators have used a definition based on residual bowel length adjusted for age. The normal length of the neonatal intestine varies markedly with gestational age. A prospective autopsy study of 30 stillborn and newborn infants varying in gestational age from 19 to 40 weeks has shown that overall intestinal length for infants between 19 and 27 weeks gestation increased from 142±22 cm to 304±44 cm for a comparable group over 35 weeks gestation [4]. Knowing that small and large bowel more than double in length during latter gestation may have value in estimating prognosis and planning treatment for many preterm SBS patients previously considered to have inadequate remaining intestine for survival [5]. For neonates operated on between 27 and 35 weeks' gestation, SBS is said to exist if the remaining bowel segment is less than 50 cm and for neonates over 35 weeks less than 72 cm [6]. In the literature, intestinal failure and short bowel are used interchangeably. In practice, although loss of small bowel is the major cause of intestinal failure, there are situations in which the gastrointestinal tract fails to nourish the individual adequately because of a combination of the loss of intestinal, gastric, and pancreatic function [7]. Fortunately, the small intestine has a large functional reserve, and 40-50% can usually be resected without major metabolic or nutritional sequelae [8]. Several reports have stated that 50% or more of expected small bowel length must be resected to produce SBS [9, 10]. Rickham reviewed his clinical experience over the last 20 years in neonates and infants with the short-gut syndrome. He defined an extensive resection as that leaving 75cm of remaining small bowel. The author notes that in this period there had been considerable development with respect to the problem. All children were kept alive by means of PN. The author concludes that further life is only possible and meaningful if the child can adapt itself to the new situation and if more than 50 cm of small intestine remains [11]. In one series of infants with SBS due to surgical resection during the neonatal period, the likelihood of achieving independence from parenteral nutrition was more than 60 percent for infants with residual small intestine length >38 cm, as compared with 7 percent in those with residual small intestine length <15 cm [12]. Several reports describe survival with a very short remnant intestine. Kurz et al described a full-term baby who underwent massive small bowel resection which left 11 cm of the proximal jejunum and was successfully weaned from total parenteral nutrition [12]. Iacono et al have described a case of extreme short bowel syndrome and review the guidelines for predicting survival in patients with very short gut [13]. The average length of the adult human small intestine is approximately 600 cm, as calculated from studies performed on cadavers. According to Lennard-Jones and to Weser, this figure ranges from 260-800 cm [14] and resection of 40-50% of the total length of the small intestine is usually well tolerated. Adults with residual small intestine of less than 180 cm are at risk for developing SBS; those with less than 60 cm of small intestine (but with a colon) are unlikely to achieve independence from parenteral nutrition [1-3]. Most adult patients with an intact duodenum, a jejunal length greater than 200 cm, and an intact colon can eventually be managed on oral intake alone. However, patients estimated to have less than 200 cm of jejunum remaining after surgery should not necessarily be excluded from an attempt at enteral feeding [15].

The problem with these definitions is that short bowel syndrome is not strictly an anatomic entity and that nutrient absorption may not correlate with length of the remaining gut. Although it is common to use intestinal remnant length in the definition of intestinal failure, particularly of SBS, the functional capability of the gut is of greater importance. Short gut syndrome is a functional rather than anatomic entity and its definition may be based on the need for intervention: patients requiring parenteral nutrition support for greater than 1 to 3 month after massive small bowel resection can be defined as having SBS [16]. The Canadian Association of Paediatric Surgeons (CAPS) defines SBS as the need for total parenteral nutrition (TPN) greater than 42 days after bowel resection, or a residual small bowel length of less than 25% expected for gestational age [17]. Balance studies performed by quantifying energy intake and fecal energy loss are perhaps the gold standard for assessing function. These studies have demonstrated that intestinal failure may be defined by measurements of wet weight and energy absorption. In general, patients who absorb less than 1.4 kg/day of wet weight or less than 4.9 MJ/day or 84% of their calculated basic energy needs according to the Harris Benedict equations depend on parenteral fluid or energy support [18]. Frequently, these are patients with less than 50–70 cm of small bowel, if the colon is in continuity, or less than 100–150 cm small bowel, if the resection is associated with a resection of ileo-colic junction [19, 20]. However, the balance studies are cumbersome. Thus, there has been continued interest in physiologic parameters to assess functional gut mass. Recently, plasma citrulline has been recommended to be a biological marker of enterocyte mass. Citrulline, an amino acid that is not incorporated into exogenous or endogenous proteins, is synthesized in enterocytes from muscle-derived glutamine and converted by the kidneys into arginine. It is believed that patients with a plasma citrulline level of 20 μmol/L or less have short bowel syndrome and require permanent home total parenteral nutrition [21]. In a study of 57 patients with nonmalignant short bowel syndrome who were followed for at least two years, a level of <20 micromol/L identified patients destined to have permanent intestinal failure with positive and negative predictive values of 95 and 86 percent, respectively [22]. A study in children with SBS demonstrated that plasma citrulline levels were strong predictors of parenteral nutrition and correlated well with a patient's recorded bowel length. A cutoff level of 15 micromol/L was found to be an accurate prognostic measure regarding the likelihood of future PN independence [23-24].

B. Incidence of Short Bowel Syndrome

In the USA, the most recent data for incidence and prevalence of SBS are from 1992. At that time, it was estimated based on extrapolated data from the Oley Foundation Home TPN Registry that approximately 40,000 patients required TPN each year in USA, and approximately 26% of these patients had short bowel syndrome [25]. However, some patients with a primary TPN indication of malignancy or radiation enteritis may have had short bowel syndrome as well. SBS affects an estimated 20,000 Americans (children and adults) [26]. The annual prevalence of home TPN has been estimated at approximately 120 per million, of whom one-quarter have SBS [27-28]. In comparison, the most recent European survey, in 1997, indicated that the incidence of home total parenteral nutrition (TPN) had remained approximately 3 per million and that the prevalence had increased to 4 per million [29]. The largest single group of patients who received home TPN were those with SBS (35%). The difference in home TPN use between the USA and Europe is likely multi-factorial and may reflect differences in the calculation of prevalence. In preliminary data from the Canadian Collaborative Short Bowel Study Group, the incidence of SBS occurring in infants and children was 4.8 per million population [3]. Previous studies regarding the need for intestinal transplantation have suggested an incidence of 2 to 3 patients per million population per year, of which typically 50% are pediatric [30,31]. A large cohort of hospitalized neonates with very low birth weight encompassing 16 tertiary neonatal centers within the United States demonstrated an incidence of SBS between 0.7% and 1.1% depending upon birth weight [27]. The Canadian Collaborative Study Group estimated the incidence of SBS across Canada as 4.8 per million population per year [32]. A study from the Province of Ontario, Canada, estimated the incidence of SBS to be 24.5 per 100,000 live births and the incidence was much greater in premature live births [33]. The mortality in this study was three times higher for SBS patients than that of a control cohort matched by underlying diagnoses.

C. Historical Overview

In the early twentieth century it was first observed that the residual intestine can undergo structural changes that result in increased surface area and enhanced nutrient absorptive capacity. In 1935, Haymond analyzed a series of 257 patients who had undergone intestinal resection and concluded that patients had near-normal bowel function with resection of one-third or less of small bowel. However, loss of greater than 50% of the small bowel was associated with short bowel syndrome [34]. As recently as the mid 1950s,

Potts suggested that most newborn infants would not survive a loss of more than 15% of the small intestine [35]. In 1957 Piling and Cresson [36] described the first successful extensive resection in two infants, who survived with only 26 and 28 cm of remaining small bowel. Subsequently, many series of patients have documented survival in infants with even shorter small bowel remnants. A review of 50 infants with significant small bowel resection showed a good probability of survival with 15cm or more of residual gut when ileocecal valve is preserved; a loss of ileocecal valve, however, requires at least 40cm of residual small bowel for a reasonable chance to survive [37].

Since the mid 1960s when Wilmore et al have described the first group of infants in whom total parenteral nutrition was used in conjunction with surgical treatment of catastrophic gastrointestinal anomalies [38,39], management of extreme short bowel syndrome has changed dramatically with notable improvements in survival and quality of life in patients with this syndrome. The series of Rickman et al in 1977 demonstrated excellent survival in children with 26 to 75 cm of small bowel and suggested 20 cm to be the critical length of remaining bowel for survival [11]. Dorney et al have described a 70% survival rate in neonates with very short small bowel (less than or equal to 38 cm jejunoileum) beginning in the first month of life who were enrolled in a home parenteral nutrition program between 1977 and 1984 [40]. Goulet has described 86 infants who had undergone resection of more than 50% of the small bowel. Patients were classified into two groups depending on the length of residual small bowel: group 1 had less than 40 cm of small bowel and group 2 had 40 to 80 cm of residual small bowel. Patients in group 2 had significantly better survival rates than those in group 1 (92.0% vs 66.6%).

The patients in group 1 who were born after 1980, when home parenteral nutrition was introduced, had better survival rates than those who were treated before 1980 (95.0% vs 65.0%) [41]. The last decade of the 20th century has seen intestinal transplantation achieve clinical applicability over a wide range of disease entities in children and adults including SBS [42]. The overall short term outcome and survival of pediatric recipients of intestinal transplantation has significantly improved over the last 2 decades and most of the long term survivors achieve enteral autonomy and good social functioning and quality of life.

D. Etiology

In pediatric population, SBS occurs in newborns and infants suffering from necrotizing enterocolitis, intestinal atresias, long-segment Hirschsprung's disease and malrotation with volvulus requiring massive intestinal resection (Table 1). In adults, the SBS, an anatomically shortened gut remnant, accounts for approximately one third of patients with intestinal failure. Extensive resection is related to mesenteric vascular accidents, malignancy, radiation strictures, adhesive obstruction and Crohn's disease. Other etiologies include trauma, fistula, scleroderma, radiation enteritis and intestinal obstruction [43-45].

Table 1. Causes of short bowel syndrome

Prenatal/Neonatal	Older children	Adults
Necrotizing enterocolitis Intestinal atresias Malrotation with volvulus Extensive agangliosis Gastroschisis Cloacal exstrophy Congenital SBS	Crohn's disease Mesenteric infarction Radiation enteritis Tumors Trauma	Crohn's disease Superior mesenteric artery thrombosis Superior mesenteric vein thrombosis Trauma Desmoid tumor Volvulus Pseudo-obstruction Massive resection secondary to tumor Radiation enteritis

In patients born with a normal gastrointestinal tract, the most frequent cause of resection is necrotizing enterocolitis (NEC), especially in premature infants. Importantly, infants with SBS following necrotizing enterocolitis have longer hospital stays than those with other etiologies. The incidence of intestinal failure among infants undergoing surgical treatment for NEC is high. Recently, 473 patients with NEC were enrolled in a multicenter prospective cohort study. Intestinal failure was defined as the requirement for parenteral nutrition for more than 90 days. Logistic regression was used to identify predictors of intestinal failure. Variables characteristic of severe NEC (low birth weight, antibiotic use, ventilator use, and greater extent of bowel resection) were associated with the development of intestinal failure [46]. Bowel-preserving strategies for NEC, designed to limit SBS, are based on peritoneal drainage, limited resection, or a combination of both. Drainage-based strategies are generally favored in smaller neonates, while laparotomy-based strategies are favored in larger patients, especially those with a more limited extent of intestinal injury [47]. Intestinal atresia may occur anywhere in the small intestine and may be either isolated or multiple. The so-called "apple peel" syndrome results from an abnormal development of the superior mesenteric artery and results commonly in short gut [48]. Patients with complex gastroschisis and intestinal anomalies have a significant risk for progression to short bowel syndrome and is a result of resection for ischemia or bowel injury [49]. Hirschsprung disease involving the small bowel as well as the colon is a cause of SBS [50]. Although intestinal aganglionosis was first reported as a cause of intestinal obstruction by Harold Hirschsprung in 1888, the first report of total intestinal aganglionosis did not occur until 1951 [51]. Thereafter, two reviews brought the world's experience to 11[52] and 12[53] cases, respectively, and the experience was extended to a 13th case in 1985. This rare entity accounts for less than 5% to 10% of all reported cases of Hirschsprung's disease, whether in the United States or in Japan [54,55]. In rare instances, the SBS may be congenital in origin, with the neonatal bowel being short in length at birth. Hasosah et al describe a term infant with congenital SBS who presented with chronic diarrhea and failure to thrive [56]. At laparotomy, the small bowel length was measured to be 50 cm from the duodenum to the ileocecal valve. The etiopathogenesis of congenital SBS is unknown and several reports have noted high mortality for these cases [57,58]. Although an upper GI small bowel follow-through can confirm the presence of malrotation and suggest short bowel length, the diagnosis of congenital SBS is typically established at surgical laparotomy. In older children, the causes of short bowel syndrome include Crohn's disease, mesenteric infarction, radiation enteritis and the loss of bowel following tumors and trauma. Several reports described a significant intestinal loss in children through transanal evisceration from sitting on unprotected swimming pool suction drains [22]. Intestinal failure can also be due to mucosal diseases (severe villous atrophy), dysmotility disorders (eg, pseudo-obstruction), severe maldigestive disorders, and other conditions [39,40].

The etiology of intestinal failure in children was changing in the last decade. Recent evidence has suggested an increasing incidence of SBS as a postoperative complication. This most commonly occurs because of repeated operations for intestinal obstruction, but it may be related to infarction secondary to vascular injury, volvulus, or hypotension [59]. Advances in management of NEC are improving survival of infants with SBS. There is now a whole generation of pediatric SBS patients who are becoming adults. Fewer patients should be undergoing aggressive resection for Crohn's disease, but SBS remains a common problem in these patients.

Conflict of Interest

None declared.

Acknowledgment

None declared.

References

[1] Booth IW, Lander AD. Short bowel syndrome. *Bailliere's Clin Gastroenterol* 1998;12:739-72.
[2] Vanderhoof JA. Short bowel syndrome. *Neonat Gastroenterol* 1996;23:377-86.
[3] Sigalet DL. Short bowel syndrome in infants and children: an overview. *Semin Pediatr Surg* 2001;10:49-55.
[4] Touloukian RJ, Smith GJW. Normal intestinal length in preterm infants. *J Pediatr Surg* 1983; 18: 720-3.
[5] Shatari T, Clark MA, Lee JR, Keighley MR. Reliability of radiographic measurement of small intestinal length. *Colorectal Dis* 2004; 6:327-9.
[6] Galea MH, Holliday H, Carachi R, Kapila L. Short-bowel syndrome: a collective review. *J Pediatr Surg* 1992; 27: 592-6.
[7] Jeejeebhoy KN. Management of short bowel syndrome: avoidance of total parenteral nutrition. *Gastroenterology.* 2006 ;130(2 Suppl 1):S60-6.
[8] Jeejeebhoy KN. Therapy of the short-gut syndrome, *Lancet* 1983; 25;1(8339):1427-30.
[9] Klish WJ, Putnam TC. The short gut. *Am J Dis Child* 1981; 135: 1056-61.

[10] Urban E, Weser E. Intestinal adaptation to bowel resection, In Stollerman GH (ed): *Advances in internal medicine,* vol 26. Chicago, Year Book Medical Publishers, Inc, 1980; pp 265-291.

[11] Rickham PP, Irving I, Shmerling DH. Long-term results following extensive small bowel resection in the neonatal period. *Prog Pediatr Surg* 1977; 10: 65-75.

[12] Quirós-Tejeira RE, Ament ME, Reyen L, Herzog F, Merjanian M, Olivares-Serrano N, Vargas JH. Long-term parenteral nutritional support and intestinal adaptation in children with short bowel syndrome: a 25-year experience. *J Pediatr* 2004;145:157-62.

[13] Kurz R, Sauer H. Treatment and metabolic findings in extreme short-bowel syndrome with 11 cm jejunal remnant. *J Pediatr Surg* 1983;18:257-63.

[14] Iacono G, Carroccio A, Montalto G, Cavataio F, Lo Cascio M, Notarbatolo A. Extreme short bowel syndrome: a case for reviewing the guidelines for predicting survival. *J Pediatr Gastroenterol Nutr* 1993;16:216-9.

[15] Weser E. Nutritional aspects of malabsorption: short gut adaptation. *Clin Gastroenterol.* 1983;12:443-61.

[16] American Gastroenterological Association. American Gastroenterological Association medical position statement: short bowel syndrome and intestinal transplantation. *Gastroenterology* 2003; 124:1105.

[17] Georgeson KE, Breaux CW. Outcome and intestinal adaptation in neonatal short bowel syndrome. *J Pediatr Surg* 1992; 27:344-50.

[18] Grant D. Intestinal transplantation: 1997 report of the international registry. Intestinal transplant registry. *Transplantation* 1999; 67:1061-4.

[19] Jeppesen PB, Mortensen PB. Intestinal failure defined by measurements of intestinal energy and wet weight absorption. *Gut* 2000;46:701-6.

[20] Carbonnel F, Cosnes J, Chevret S, Beaugerie L, Ngo Y, Malafosse M, Parc R, Le Quintrec Y, Gendre JP. The role of anatomic factors in nutritional autonomy after extensive small bowel resection. *JPEN J Parenter Enteral Nutr* 1996;20:275-80.

[21] Nightingale JM, Lennard Jones JE, Walker ER, Farthing MJ. Jejunal efflux in short bowel syndrome (see comments). *Lancet* 1990; 336: 765-8.

[22] Crenn P, Coudray-Lucas C, Thuillier F, Cynober L, Messing B. Postabsorptive plasma citrulline concentration is a marker of absorptive

enterocyte mass and intestinal failure in humans. *Gastroenterology* 2000; 119:1496-05.

[23] Santarpia L, Catanzano F, Ruoppolo M, et al. Citrulline blood levels as indicators of residual intestinal absorption in patients with short bowel syndrome. *Ann Nutr Metab* 2008; 53:137.

[24] Fitzgibbons S, Ching YA, Valim C. Relationship between serum citrulline levels and progression to parenteral nutrition independence in children with short bowel syndrome. *J Pediatr Surg* 2009; 44:928.

[25] Oley Foundation. North American home parenteral and enteral nutrition patient registry annual report, 1994.

[26] Cole CR, Hansen NI, Higgins RD. Very low birth weight preterm infants with surgical short bowel syndrome: incidence, morbidity and mortality, and growth outcomes at 18 to 22 months. *Pediatrics* 2008; 122; e573-82/

[27] Howard L, Ament M, Fleming CR, Shike M, Steiger E. Current use and clinical outcome of home parenteral and enteral nutrition therapies in the Unated States. *Gastroenterology* 1995; 109: 355-65.

[28] Howard L, Ament M, Fleming CR. Four years of North American registry home parenteral nutrition outcome data and their implications for patient management. JPEN 1991; 15:384-93.Koeberle E. Resection de deux meters d'intestin grele. *Bull Acad Med* 1881; 8:249-50.

[29] Van Gossum A, Bakker H, Bozetti F, et al. Home parenteral nutrition in adults: a European multicentre study in 1997. *Clin Nutr* 1999;18:135–140.

[30] Grant D. Intestinal transplantation: 1197 report of the international registry. *Transplantation* 1999; 67: 1061-4.

[31] Abu-Elmagd K, Reyes J. Factors impacting the survival of children with intestinal failure referred for intestinal transplantation. *J Pediatr Surg* 1999; 34:27-32.

[32] Canadian Collaborative Study Group Protocol: CAPS Web Page, http:/www.caps.ca, Accessed Nov 16, 1999.

[33] Wales PW, de Silva N, Kim J. Neonatal short bowel syndrome: population-based estimates of incidence and mortality rates. *J Pediatr Surg* 2004, 39, 690-5.

[34] Haymond H E. Massive resection of the small intestine. *Surg Gynecol Obstet* 1935;51: 693-705.

[35] Potts WJ. Pediatric surgery. *J Am Med Assoc* 1955; 157: 627-30.

[36] Pilling GP, Cresson SL. Massive resection of small intestine in the neonatal period. Report of two successful cases and review of the literature. *Pediatrics* 1957; 19: 940-8.

[37] Galea MH, Holliday H, Carachi R, Kapila L. Short-bowel syndrome: a collective review. *J Pediatr Surg* 1992;27: 592-6.

[38] Wilmore DW. Factors correlating with a successful outcome following extensive intestinal resection in the newborn infant. *J Pediatr* 1972; 80: 88-93.

[39] Wilmore DW, Groff DB, Bishop HC, Dudrick SJ. Total parenteral nutrition in infants with catastrophic gastrointestinal anomalies. *J Pediatr Surg* 1969; 4: 181-189.

[40] Dorney SF, Ament ME, Berquist WE, Vargas JH, Hassall E. Improved survival in very short small bowel of infancy with use of long-term parenteral nutrition. *J Pediatr* 1985; 107:521-5.

[41] Goulet OJ, Revillon Y, Jan D, De Potter S, Maurage C, Lortat-Jacob S, Martelli H, Nihoul-Fekete C, Ricour C. Neonatal short bowel syndrome. *J Pediatr* 1991;119 (1 Pt 1):18-23.

[42] Reyes J. Intestinal transplantation for children with short bowel syndrome. *Sem Pediatr Surg* 2001; 10:99-104.

[43] DiBaise JK, Young RJ, Vanderhoof JA. Intestinal rehabilitation and the short bowel syndrome. *Am J Gastroenterol* 2004; 99:1386-95.

[44] Sturm A, Layer P, Goebell H. Short-bowel syndrome: an update on the therapeutic approach. *Scand J Gastroenterol* 1997; 32:289-96.

[45] Thompson JS. Inflammatory disease and outcome of short bowel syndrome. *Am J Surg* 2000; 180:551–5.

[46] Duro D, Kalish LA, Johnston P, Jaksic T, McCarthy M, Martin C, Dunn JC, Brandt M, Nobuhara KK, Sylvester KG, Moss RL, Duggan C. Risk factors for intestinal failure in infants with necrotizing enterocolitis: a Glaser Pediatric Research Network study. *J Pediatr.* 2010; 157:203-8.

[47] Petty JK, Ziegler MM. Operative strategies for necrotizing enterocolitis: The prevention and treatment of short-bowel syndrome. *Semin Pediatr Surg* 2005; 14:191-8.

[48] Goulet O, Baglin-Gobet S, Jais JP, Michel JL, Jan D, Ricour C. Outcome and long-term growth after extensive small bowel resection in the neonatal period: a survey of 87 children. *Eur J Pediatr Surg* 2005;15:95–101.

[49] Salihu HM, Aliyu ZY, Pierre-Louis BJ, Obuseh FA, Druschel CM, Kirby RS. Omphalocele and gastroschisis: black-white disparity in infant survival. *Birth Defects Res A Clin Mol Teratol* 2004; 70:586-91.

[50] Hackam DJ, Reblock KK, Redlinger RE, Barksdale EM. Diagnosis and outcome of Hirschsprung's disease: does age really matter? *Pediatr Surg Int* 2004;20: 319-22.

[51] Bodian M, Carter CO, Ward BCH. Hirschsprung's disease. *Lancet* 1951; 1:302-4.

[52] Talwalker UC. Aganglionosis of the entire bowel. *J Pediatr Surg* 1976; 11:213-6.

[53] Saperstein L, Pollack J, Beck AR. Total intestinal aganglionosis. *Mt Sinai J Med* 1980; 47:72-3.

[54] Kleinhaus S, Boley SJ, Sheran M, Sieber WK. Hirschsprung's disease: a survey ofthe members of the surgical section of the American Academy of Pediatrics. *J Pediatr Surg* 1979; 14:588-97.

[55] Ikeda K, Goto S. Diagnosis and treatment of Hirschsprung's disease in Japan. *Ann Surg* 1984; 199:400-5.

[56] Hasosah M, Lemberg DA, Skarsgard E, Schreiber R. Congenital short bowel syndrome: a case report and review of the literature. *Can J Gastroenterol* 2008;22:71-4.

[57] Erez I, Reish O, Kovalivker M, Lazar L, Raz A, Katz S. Congenital short-bowel and malrotation: Clinical presentation and outcome of six affected offspring in three related families. *Eur J Pediatr Surg* 2001;11:331-4.

[58] Kern IB, Leece A, Bohane T. Congenital short gut, malrotation, and dysmotility of the small bowel. *J Pediatr Gastroenterol Nutr* 1990;11:411-5.

[59] Goulet O, Sauvat F, Ruemmele F, Caldari D, Damotte D, Cezard JP, Lacaille F, Canioni D, Hugot JP, Berebi D, Sarnacki S, Colomb V, Jan D, Aigrain Y, Revillon Y. Results of the Paris program: ten years of pediatric intestinal transplantation. *Transplant Proc* 2005; 37:1667-70.

In: Short Bowel Syndrome in Children
Editor: Igor Sukhotnik
ISBN: 978-1-62948-518-8

Chapter II

Survival Outcomes of Pediatric Intestinal Failure Patients and the Cost of Comprehensive Care

Matthew W. Ralls, M.D., Meghan A. Arnold, M.D. and Daniel H. Teitelbaum*, M.D.
C.S. Mott Children's Hospital,
University of Michigan Hospital and Health Systems.
Ann Arbor, MI, US

Abstract

Intestinal failure (IF) affects 40,000 or approximately 0.2-4.9 per million individuals a year [1], encompassing both adult and pediatric patients. This devastating disease process comprises immense consequences for patients and their family, as well as the medical community as a whole. Insufficient intestinal absorptive capacity is a difficult medical dilemma. Therapies employed in the treatment of these individuals carry significant risk of complications as well. The overall

* Address correspondence to: Daniel H. Teitelbaum, M.D.; Section of Pediatric Surgery, University of Michigan; CS Mott Children's Hospital; 1540 E. Hospital Dr., SPC 4211, Ann Arbor, MI 48109-4211; Phone: +1-734-936-8464. Fax: +1-734-936-9784. E-mail: dttlbm@umich.edu.

mortality for pediatric IF patients has been reported to approach 25 to 30% in reviews [3]. However, over the past decade has shown several exciting improvements in the care of IF patients, with many centers now showing markedly improved survival. The financial toll of IF is significant and can exceed an average of more than $1.5 million [3] for the first few years of life with each readmission to the hospital averaging over $250,000 [4,5].

Overcoming caloric deficiencies and meeting specific nutrient needs are the primary objectives in caring for these patients. Difficulties in the management of patients with IF result not only from the underlying disease processes, but also the complications that arise from treatment strategies. Improper disease management can leave the patient with inadequate energy substrates for normal growth and at risk for developing nutrient deficiencies leading to their downstream complications. The need for supplemental or total parenteral nutrition (PN) is often required to sustain normal growth, development and an ideal nutritional status. While certainly beneficial and necessary, numerous complications are associated with the PN therapy and the central access devices needed for its delivery. These complications including blood stream infection, venous thrombosis, metabolic derangements, anemia, hepatic dysfunction bone demineralization and renal stones.

I. Outcomes

The diversity of the disease processes which lead to IF and their wide range of complications makes the complexity of patient care in this population immense. Multiple studies had reported an overall mortality rate ranging from 16% to nearly 40% in some previous series [6]. More recently, however, groups have shown a dramatic increase in survival. Hess et al demonstrated a decrease in mortality from 30% to 6.6% over the past two decades (Figure 1) [7].

Using a multivariate analysis approach the one factor which contributed most significantly to this marked improvement in survival was the implementation of a comprehensive multispecialty care team. Other groups have reported similar improved survival rates ranging from 87% to 100% in recent years; although the precise factor which has driven this marked improvement is not precisely known [8-10]. While not universally accepted as the cause of improved survival [11], a multidisciplinary group including surgeons, gastroenterologists, nutritionists, pharmacists and specialized nurses has the advantage of input from many specialists at every point of care. In addition the patient population is small enough for the members of this team to have an intimate knowledge of the individuals' disease processes and details of each case allowing for more rapid responses to issues as they arise. Moreover, with experience, the group can establish protocols for enteral and parenteral nutrition, standardize laboratory testing and provide continuity and long-term monitoring of outcomes. A multidisciplinary approach helps make the enormity of managing this population more practical.

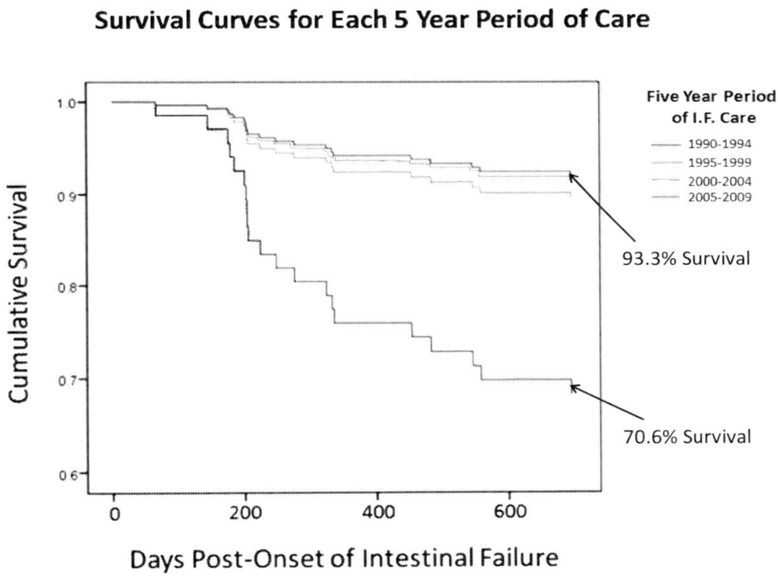

Figure 1. Survival outcomes from a single intestinal failure clinical program over two decades. Note the progressive improved survival over time. Data derived from Hess, et al, J Surg Res. 2011 [7].

A. Nutrition

This multidisciplinary team can impact specific therapies but enteral autonomy (i.e., weaning from PN) is the primary target for treatment. While the composition of PN and enteral nutrition is beyond the scope of this chapter there have been great advances in nutrition and in the care of patients requiring nutritional support over the last several years [12-14]. While intestinal failure encompasses a number of disorders, the prevalent condition is short bowel syndrome (SBS) which can be broken down into three phases which describe the physiologic derangements in these patients which directly leads to how they are managed medically. Nutritional goals during these phases must be tailored to each individual, but the overarching themes are similar across all patients. The acute phase, which occurs in the immediate postoperative period, is marked by poor absorption of all luminal contents [15]. Aggressive monitoring is necessary to quickly correct any electrolyte imbalances that arise and fluid shifts that could lead to hemodynamic instability [16]. The adaptation phase follows next and can last for two years or longer [17]. This phase is characterized by a period of intestinal morphologic changes that can result in enteral autonomy. During this period there is more stability in nutritional requirements but continual adjustments are necessary to meet the physiologic demands of the growing child. The last phase, maintenance, occurs when the maximal absorptive capacity of the bowel has been reached and no further intrinsic changes will increase the likelihood of weaning from PN [18]. It is during this phase that treatments such as bowel lengthening, administration of growth factors or bowel transplantation may result in the ability to wean from PN. While a number of factors contribute to a child's ability to wean from PN, the length of intestine has often been cited as the major factor. One of the great confounders in understanding the contribution of intestinal length to the ability to wean from PN, however, it is the fact that many children undergo a significant bowel resection early in life after which point further intestinal lengthening occurs spontaneously as the child grows. This is particularly evident when the child is born prematurely, as measurements of infants undergoing intestinal surgery in the first few years of life show that the intestine lengthens exponentially during the third trimester [19]. To address this problem, Spencer et al advocating describing the true intestinal length as the percent predicted of the expected intestinal length at any gestational age. This has led to a wide stratification of outcomes based on children with 10% or more of predicted small bowel length compared to those with less than 10% of predicted length (Figure 2). This stratification can be helpful in providing guidance to families about their child's overall prognosis.

Another key factor which is useful in predicting the likelihood of enteral autonomy is the function of the small bowel itself. Almost 20 years ago Cynober identified citrulline is an amino acid which was produced predominately by intestinal epithelial cells [30]. Subsequent data has shown that higher levels of citrulline are associated with a greater ability to wean from PN, and that levels below 20 micromol/L were associated with a poor chance of weaning from TPN [21]. Recently Wales et al have shown that intestinal lengthening procedures lead to increased citrulline values [22]; this may be one of the key mechanisms by which intestinal lengthening contributes to intestinal autonomy.

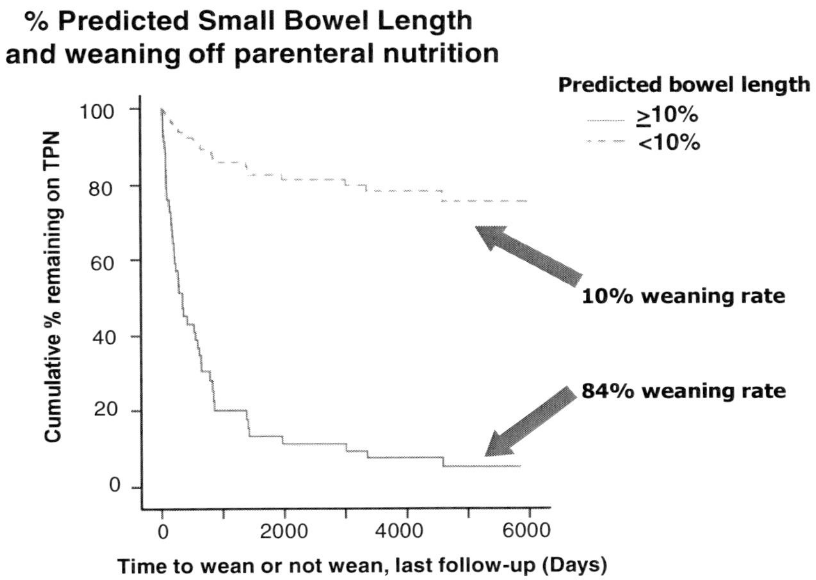

Figure 2. Ability to successfully wean off of TPN. Shown are the % predicted small bowel length and the likelihood of weaning off parenteral nutrition as stratified by patients with≥10% predicted small bowel length for their gestational age compared to those with <10% predicted length. Note the dramatic differences in success in weaning. Derived from Spencer, et al, Ann Surg, 2005 [6].

B. PN-Associated Liver Disease

Prolonged PN administration predictably results in PN-associated liver disease which, at its most extreme, leads to hepatic fibrosis and liver failure [23]. The etiology of this hepatic dysfunction is multifactorial and includes direct toxic effects, impaired bile drainage and an imbalance of carbohydrate and lipids. While there are suspected direct toxic effect of amino acids, another important etiologic factor is a breakdown in the intestinal barrier function which leads to bacterial translocation into the portal venous system [24]. This was recently illustrated in a mouse model of TPN and appears to be mediated by increased Toll-like receptor 4 signaling [25], potentially due to the development of an aberrant microbiome as a result of TPN administration [26]. An additional contributing factor the development of PN-associated liver disease may result from the down-regulation of several hepatocyte transporters critical for moving bile components out of hepatocytes [27]. Failure of bile drainage results in direct hepatotoxicity. The imbalance of carbohydrates and lipids from physiologic levels can lead to steatohepatitis, intrahepatic cholestasis and fibrosis which all culminate in liver failure [18]. Targeted measures that alleviate liver-related complications have been shown to lead to dramatic improvements in overall survival [10]. These therapies include early enteral feeding [28], antibiotic prophylaxis for intestinal bacterial overgrowth [29], fish-oil based lipids [30-32] and intestinal lengthening procedures [33]. Our understanding of the implications of the type and dose of the lipid component of PN has recently been extensively examined. Two recent publications have suggested that a reduction in the dose of soybean-based lipids from 3 g/kg/day to either 1 g/kg/day or 1 g/kg given twice a week resulted in a slower rise in direct bilirubin values and, therefore, a lower incidence of PN-associated cholestasis [34-35]. Future work is needed to establish the optimal soybean-based lipid dose which both minimizes the development of cholestasis but allows for adequate growth, particularly in the neonatal population. A decrease in the incidence of severe liver disease has resulted in a marked improvement in patient survival and overall outcomes.

C. Central Venous Access Devices

A major morbidity associated with PN administration is catheter-related blood stream infection (CRBSI) [36]. The incidence is reported between 16,000 and 500,000 adult cases annually in the US [37]. CRBSI results in significant morbidity and mortality in children with intestinal failure and add significantly to health care costs with each episode costing on average$35,000 per event [38]. Catheter locks (antibiotic or ethanol) have led to a dramatic decline the incidence of CRBSI in high-risk IF children [39-41]. In fact, the CDC now recommends the use of prophylactic antimicrobial lock solutions in any patient with a history of multiple CRBSI [42]. While somewhat newer, ethanol lock therapy has resulted in a 10-fold decline in CRBSI rates; including those due to fungi [39,43]. Most recently, ethanol lock therapy has been used to treat CRBSI and has resulted in the salvage of intravenous lines which had failed conventional antibiotic therapy [44].

D. Intestinal Lengthening Procedures

The ability to wean from PN is strongly correlated with bowel length [45]. Surgical procedures to increase intestinal length, therefore, have been practiced for years. The Bianchi procedure, a longitudinal division of a dilated intestinal lumen followed by 3 anastomoses to re-establish intestinal continuity, has largely been replaced by the serial transverse enteroplasty procedure (STEP). The STEP procedure was first described by Kim and Jaksic in 2003 [46] and involves a series of alternating V-shaped staple lines along the length of dilated segment of bowel. The benefits of the STEP procedure include its ability to increase bowel length and decrease bowel diameter without the need for numerous anastomoses. Initially, a STEP procedure was recommended when bowel was sufficiently dilated and a relative plateau of intestinal adaptation had been reached (i.e. no longer able to advance enteral feeds). Recently, however, evidence suggests that earlier intervention may lead to better overall outcomes [47]. Alternative methods for intestinal lengthening are being developed, but primarily exist in the research realm. Mechanotransduction to induce longitudinal intestinal growth is currently being studied [48] as is the use of intestinal enteroids improve absorptive surface area [49]. Because both of these novel methods are years away from clinical testing, the STEP procedure continues to be the most common lengthening option utilized. All patients with PN dependence should be considered for surgical lengthening; however, those with evidence of progressive hepatic dysfunction should be referred for intestinal transplantation [50].

E. Intestinal Transplantation

Indications for intestinal transplantation include liver dysfunction, loss of major venous access, frequent central line-related sepsis or recurrent episodes of severe dehydration despite intravenous fluid management [51]. Once the decision for transplantation has been made the care team must decide which organs to transplant – liver alone, liver with small bowel or multivisceral (stomach, duodenum, pancreas, liver and small bowel). A recent large review found that the 5 year actuarial survival of children transplanted between 1985 and 2009 was approximately 50% and has remained relatively stable over time [14]. For adults, although survival trends are improving somewhat, the 5 year survival is still ranges from 43 to 75% [52].

II. Cost

With the advent of parenteral nutrition and bowel lengthening procedures survival has greatly improved over the past few decades for pediatric SBS patients. These patients continue to have chronic medical needs, however, which have resulted in a significant cost burden for the health care system. One of the earliest reports of the cost of home PN was published by Burnes et al in 1992 who analyzed data involving 63 patients including some as young as 11 years of age [53]. During the 3 years that patients were followed 73% required at least one hospitalization with a mean hospital stay of 10.6 days. Fewer than half required more than 1 admission. More than two-thirds of the admissions were for suspected catheter sepsis illustrating the importance of preventing this complication through proper aseptic techniques. The cost of home PN is variable in the literature and has steadily increased over time coincident with health care costs overall. In the early 1980s annual home PN cost was estimated at only $20,000 but these costs had increased to almost $100,000 annually about20 years ago [54], and up to $200,000 dollars by 1998 [55]. Direct costs related to home PN therapy include the solution itself as well as durable medical equipment needed for its administration. The overall cost of care has continued to climb and is now estimated to be between $238 and $390 per day according to Medicare data [56]. Medicare reimbursements are adjusted quarterly; data available most recently for the state of Michigan is shown in Table 1. Not included in these costs are outpatient clinic visits, laboratory tests and time missed from work. Despite its cost, however, home PN administration is 50-75% less expensive than obtaining the same nutrition therapy while hospitalized.

Table 1. Current Medicare Reimbursement for Home Parenteral Nutrition, by Component

Component	Fee
Lipid	$12.63 per 10g
10 to 51g Protein	$199.85
52 to 73g Protein	$258.25
74 to 100g Protein	$314.40

Adapted from National Government Services, Inc. DME MAC Jurisdiction B 3rd Quarter 2013 DMEPOS/PEN Fee Schedule found athttp://tinyurl.com/kena39p.

Numerous groups have postulated intestinal transplantation may actually reduce the cost of care for SBS patients since the initial expense of the transplant procedure is offset by no longer needing to be on prolonged PN therapy [57]. According to Sudan's analysis the cost of various intestinal transplant procedures ranged from $132,000 to $207,000 at two major medical centers in the United States [58]. Despite the additional costs required for lifelong immunosuppression as well as hospital readmission for transplant related complications, intestinal transplantation may be cost-effective compared to prolonged PN when graft function persists beyond 1-3 years [59]. The total cost of care is less in transplant patients after two years compared to those continuing on home PN. While less expensive, the overall survival of transplantation, as described above, is not improving to the same rate as patients receiving conservative management. The cost of home care is well justified. Not only in that it is cost-savings when compared within patient care, but it allows for patients to be in their home environment. This will greatly affect quality of life. While these points are difficult to measure, Puntis describes that psychomotor delay of infants reverses shortly after discharge and that most adolescents able to enjoy a normal social life [5].

More recently a more comprehensive assessment of the cost of care has been done by studying a cohort of children with short bowel syndrome who received their inpatient, outpatient and home care within a single health system. This report estimated the average overall cost of care in the first five years after diagnosis at 1.62 ± 1.03million US dollars although costs were disproportionately high in the first year of the diagnosis [3]. The duration of the initial hospitalization averaged 67.1 ± 50.3 days in this cohort which corresponded to an average cost of care in the first year of over $505,000. Most continued expense (82%) [59] is attributed to inpatient readmissions, which are quite common in SBS patients and are often related to central line or infectious complications. In this cohort patients required 5.8 ± 3.4 readmissions to this hospital in the first year after diagnosis; each hospitalization had an average length of stay of 10.0 ± 14.7 days. In-hospital days in the first year following diagnosis averaged 119 ± 61 days per patient. The frequency of readmissions however, steadily decreased with time although overall charges remained relatively static from years 2 through 5. The total cost of care must include the sum of inpatient and home-care charges. Several millions of dollars are spent on the 40,000 adults and children receiving home PN each year [60]. As patients are living longer, home nutrition costs coupled with specialized nursing visits, laboratory studies and outpatient appointments all contribute to the significant health care expenditures required for this population. In contrast to the downward trend of inpatient costs during the first 5 years of care, home-care costs rise each year (Figure 3) [61]. Home-care charges include antimicrobials, injectables, intravenous hydration, enteral and parenteral nutrition. While these high home-care costs largely accounted for by the cost of the PN solution itself antimicrobials also contribute significantly to the expense. Interestingly, the rise in home-care charges occurs despite the fact that a majority of infants with SBS wean from PN during this time period. Home care averages $87,932 ±70,079 for the first year, but rises to $184,520±111,075 by year 5.

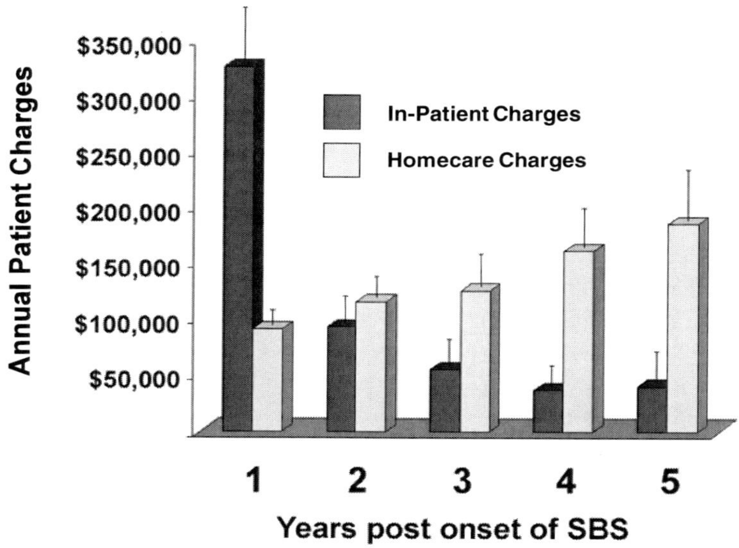

Figure 3. Total charges (in U.S. dollars corrected to the year 2005) for inpatient and outpatient clinical care of pediatric SBS patients. Note that dominant charges come from inpatient care in the first year followed by a progressive increase in outpatient costs over the next four years. Data derived from Spencer, et al, Am J Clin Nutr, 2008 [64].

Many factors contribute to variability in cost between patients. Non-survivors have been found to have increased costs at all-time points compared to survivors [2]. However, regression analysis showed that non-survival and cholestasis were not significant predictors of increased cost[2].This is somewhat counterintuitive as these two outcome measures correlate with case complexity and are therefore expected to increase cost. Other factors thought to influence disease complexity such as the etiology of SBS, presence or absence of ileocecal valve and number of septic episodes showed no significant correlation. Only bowel length (those with less than 10% of expected length) was found to independently correlate with a higher cost of care. This holds true even when non-survivors were removed from analysis [2], and may reflect a far more complex and challenging group of children.

The development of new therapies in the care of intestinal failure will impact costs much like the development of PN did in the 1970s. A promising new drug currently being investigated in the treatment of intestinal failure is teduglutide, a long-acting glucagon-like peptide-2 analog which promotes intestinal mucosal growth [62]. While the cost of this daily therapy will vary across the world one early estimate is that it will cost in excess of $300,000 per year per US patient. While some patients have successfully weaned off PN following therapy with teduglutide, many continue to need at least some PN support. In addition, the finding that a progressive decline in BMI occurs after the drug is stopped implies that some individuals might need the drug indefinitely with a concomitant neutral or negative impact on the overall cost of care (loss of the cost of PN but continued need for GLP-2) [63].

The care of patients with intestinal failure and short bowel syndrome was revolutionized with the development of parenteral nutrition. The lifetime costs of this care, however, are significant and are differentially due to inpatient and outpatient care as the individual ages. Costs for such care can be a substantial financial burden to the patients' families and insurance providers and must be considered in the overall care of this patient population.

References

[1] Colomb V, Goulet O, Ricour C. Home enteral and parenteral nutrition in children. *Baillieres Clin Gastroenterol.* Dec 1998;12(4):877-894.

[2] Squires RH, Duggan C, Teitelbaum DH, et al. Natural history of pediatric intestinal failure: initial report from the Pediatric Intestinal Failure Consortium. *J Pediatr.* Oct 2012;161(4):723-728 e722.

[3] Spencer AU, Kovacevich D, McKinney-Barnett M, et al. Pediatric short-bowel syndrome: the cost of comprehensive care. *American Journal of Clinical Nutrition.* Dec 2008;88(6):1552-1559.

[4] Ralls MW, Blackwood RA, Arnold MA, Partipilo ML, Dimond J, Teitelbaum DH. Drug Shortage-Associated Increase in Catheter-Related

Blood Stream Infection in Children. *Pediatrics.* Nov 2012;130(5):E1369-E1373.

[5] Puntis JW. The economics of home parenteral nutrition. *Nutrition.* Oct 1998;14(10):809-812.

[6] Spencer A, Safran J, Neeaga A, Brown P, Btaiche I, Teitelbaum D. Mortality and Outcomes of Pediatric Short Bowel Syndrome: Redefining Predictors of Success. *Annals of Surgery.* 2005;242:1-10.

[7] Hess RA, Welch KB, Brown PI, Teitelbaum DH. Survival outcomes of pediatric intestinal failure patients: analysis of factors contributing to improved survival over the past two decades. *Journal of Surgical Research.* Sep 2011;170(1):27-31.

[8] Nucci A, Burns RC, Armah T, et al. Interdisciplinary management of pediatric intestinal failure: a 10-year review of rehabilitation and transplantation. *J Gastrointest Surg.* Mar 2008;12(3):429-435; discussion 435-426.

[9] Pironi L, Joly F, Forbes A, et al. Long-term follow-up of patients on home parenteral nutrition in Europe: implications for intestinal transplantation. *Gut.* Jan 2011;60(1):17-25.

[10] Sigalet D, Boctor D, Robertson M, et al. Improved outcomes in paediatric intestinal failure with aggressive prevention of liver disease. *European Journal of Pediatric Surgery.* Dec 2009;19(6):348-353.

[11] Diamond IR, de Silva N, Pencharz PB, Kim JH, Wales PW. Neonatal short bowel syndrome outcomes after the establishment of the first Canadian multidisciplinary intestinal rehabilitation program: preliminary experience. *Journal of Pediatric Surgery.* May 2007;42(5):806-811.

[12] Matarese LE. Nutrition and fluid optimization for patients with short bowel syndrome. *JPEN J Parenter Enteral Nutr.* Mar 2013;37(2):161-170.

[13] Torres C, Sudan D, Vanderhoof J, et al. Role of an intestinal rehabilitation program in the treatment of advanced intestinal failure. *J Pediatr Gastroenterol Nutr.* Aug 2007;45(2):204-212.

[14] Mazariegos GV, Superina R, Rudolph J, et al. Current status of pediatric intestinal failure, rehabilitation, and transplantation: summary of a colloquium. *Transplantation.* Dec 15 2011;92(11):1173-1180.

[15] Dudrick SJ, Latifi R, Fosnocht DE. Management of the short-bowel syndrome. *Surg Clin North Am.* Jun 1991;71(3):625-643.

[16] Berger DL, Malt RA. Management of the short gut syndrome. *Adv Surg.* 1996;29:43-57.

[17] Ziegler MM. Short bowel syndrome: remedial features that influence outcome and the duration of parenteral nutrition. *J Pediatr.* Sep 1997;131(3):335-336.

[18] Sundaram A, Koutkia P, Apovian CM. Nutritional management of short bowel syndrome in adults. *J Clin Gastroenterol.* Mar 2002;34(3):207-220.

[19] Struijs MC, Diamond IR, de Silva N, Wales PW. Establishing norms for intestinal length in children. *J Pediatr Surg.* May 2009;44(5):933-938.

[20] Crenn P, Coudray-Lucas C, Thuillier F, Cynober L, Messing B. Postabsorptive plasma citrulline concentration is a marker of absorptive enterocyte mass and intestinal failure in humans. *Gastroenterology.* Dec 2000;119(6):1496-1505.

[21] Crenn P, Coudray-Lucas C, Cynober L, Messing B. Post-absorptive plasma citrulline concentration: a marker of intestinal failure in humans. *Transplantation Proceedings.* 1998;30(6):2528.

[22] Oliveira C, de Silva N, Wales PW. Five-year outcomes after serial transverse enteroplasty in children with short bowel syndrome. *J Pediatr Surg.* May 2012;47(5):931-937.

[23] Kelly DA. Liver complications of pediatric parenteral nutrition--epidemiology. *Nutrition.* Jan 1998;14(1):153-157.

[24] Stoidis CN, Misiakos EP, Patapis P, Fotiadis CI, Spyropoulos BG. Potential benefits of pro- and prebiotics on intestinal mucosal immunity and intestinal barrier in short bowel syndrome. *Nutr Res Rev.* Oct 21 2010:1-9.

[25] El Kasmi KC, Anderson AL, Devereaux MW, et al. Toll-like receptor 4-dependent Kupffer cell activation and liver injury in a novel mouse model of parenteral nutrition and intestinal injury. *Hepatology.* May 2012;55(5):1518-1528.

[26] Miyasaka EA, Feng Y, Poroyko V, et al. Total Parenteral Nutrition-Associated Lamina Propria Inflammation in Mice Is Mediated by a MyD88-Dependent Mechanism. *J Immunol.* Jun 15 2013;190(12):6607-6615.

[27] Tazuke Y, Teitelbaum DH. Alteration of canalicular transporters in a mouse model of total parenteral nutrition. *J Pediatr Gastroenterol Nutr.* Feb 2009;48(2):193-202.

[28] Nehra D, Fallon EM, Puder M. The prevention and treatment of intestinal failure-associated liver disease in neonates and children. *Surg Clin North Am.* Jun 2011;91(3):543-563.

[29] Sigalet D, Boctor D, Brindle M, Lam V, Robertson M. Elements of successful intestinal rehabilitation. *Journal of Pediatric Surgery*. Jan 2011;46(1):150-156.

[30] Burns DL, Gill BM. Reversal of parenteral nutrition-associated liver disease with a fish oil-based lipid emulsion (omegaven) in an adult dependent on home parenteral nutrition. *JPEN J Parenter Enteral Nutr*. Mar 2013;37(2):274-280.

[31] Ekema G, Falchetti D, Boroni G, et al. Reversal of severe parenteral nutrition-associated liver disease in an infant with short bowel syndrome using parenteral fish oil (Omega-3 fatty acids). *Journal of Pediatric Surgery*. Jun 2008;43(6):1191-1195.

[32] Gura KM, Duggan CP, Collier SB, et al. Reversal of parenteral nutrition-associated liver disease in two infants with short bowel syndrome using parenteral fish oil: implications for future management. *Pediatrics*. Jul 2006;118(1):e197-201.

[33] Goulet O, Ruemmele F. Causes and management of intestinal failure in children. *Gastroenterology*. Feb 2006;130(2 Suppl 1):S16-28.

[34] Rollins MD, Ward RM, Jackson WD, et al. Effect of decreased parenteral soybean lipid emulsion on hepatic function in infants at risk for parenteral nutrition-associated liver disease: A pilot study. *J Pediatr Surg*. Jun 2013;48(6):1348-1356.

[35] Cober MP, Killu G, Brattain A, Welch KB, Kunisaki SM, Teitelbaum DH. Intravenous fat emulsions reduction for patients with parenteral nutrition-associated liver disease. *J Pediatr*. Mar 2012;160(3):421-427.

[36] Rodriguez-Paz JM, Pronovost P. Prevention of catheter-related bloodstream infections. *Adv Surg*. 2008;42:229-248.

[37] Maki DG, Kluger DM, Crnich CJ. The risk of bloodstream infection in adults with different intravascular devices: a systematic review of 200 published prospective studies. *Mayo Clin Proc*. Sep 2006;81(9):1159-1171.

[38] O'Grady NP, Alexander M, Burns LA, et al. Guidelines for the prevention of intravascular catheter-related infections. *Clin Infect Dis*. May 2011;52(9):e162-193.

[39] Cober MP, Kovacevich DS, Teitelbaum DH. Ethanol-lock therapy for the prevention of central venous access device infections in pediatric patients with intestinal failure. *JPEN J Parenter Enteral Nutr*. Jan-Feb 2011;35(1):67-73.

[40] Mouw E, Chessman K, Lesher A, Tagge E. Use of an ethanol lock to prevent catheter-related infections in children with short bowel syndrome. *J Pediatr Surg.* Jun 2008;43(6):1025-1029.

[41] Sanders J, Pithie A, Ganly P, et al. A prospective double-blind randomized trial comparing intraluminal ethanol with heparinized saline for the prevention of catheter-associated bloodstream infection in immunosuppressed haematology patients. *J Antimicrob Chemother.* Oct 2008;62(4):809-815.

[42] O'Grady NP, Alexander M, Burns LA, et al. Guidelines for the prevention of intravascular catheter-related infections. *Am J Infect Control.* May 2011;39(4 Suppl 1):S1-34.

[43] Blackwood RA, Klein KC, Micel LN, et al. Ethanol Locks Therapy for Resolution of Fungal Catheter Infections. *Pediatr Infect Dis J.* Aug 12 2011.

[44] Valentine KM. Ethanol lock therapy for catheter-associated blood stream infections in a pediatric intensive care unit. *Pediatr Crit Care Med.* Nov 2011;12(6):e292-296.

[45] Spencer AU, Neaga A, West B, et al. Pediatric short bowel syndrome: redefining predictors of success. *Annals of Surgery.* Sep 2005; 242(3):403-409; discussion 409-412.

[46] Kim HB, Fauza D, Garza J, Oh JT, Nurko S, Jaksic T. Serial transverse enteroplasty (STEP): a novel bowel lengthening procedure. *Journal of Pediatric Surgery.* Mar 2003;38(3):425-429.

[47] Wood SJ, Khalil B, Fusaro F, Folaranmi SE, Sparks SA, Morabito A. Early Structured Surgical Management Plan for Neonates with Short Bowel Syndrome May Improve Outcomes. *World J Surg.* Mar 29 2013.

[48] Koga H, Sun X, Yang H, et al. Distraction-induced intestinal enterogenesis: preservation of intestinal function and lengthening after reimplantation into normal jejunum. *Ann Surg.* Feb 2012;255(2):302-310.

[49] Spurrier RG, Grikscheit TC. Tissue engineering the small intestine. *Clin Gastroenterol Hepatol.* Apr 2013;11(4):354-358.

[50] Thompson J, Sudan D. Intestinal lengthening for short bowel syndrome. *Adv Surg.* 2008;42:49-61.

[51] Mazariegos GV, Squires RH, Sindhi RK. Current perspectives on pediatric intestinal transplantation. *Curr Gastroenterol Rep.* Jun 2009;11(3):226-233.

[52] Trevizol AP, David AI, Dias ER, Mantovani D, Pecora R, D'Albuquerque LA. Intestinal and multivisceral transplantation

immunosuppression protocols--literature review. *Transplant Proc.* Oct 2012;44(8):2445-2448.

[53] Burnes JU, O'Keefe SJ, Fleming CR, Devine RM, Berkner S, Herrick L. Home parenteral nutrition--a 3-year analysis of clinical and laboratory monitoring. *JPEN J Parenter Enteral Nutr.* Jul-Aug 1992;16(4):327-332.

[54] Colomb V, Jobert-Giraud A, Lacaille F, et al. Role of lipid emulsions in cholestasis associated with long-term parenteral nutrition in children. *JPEN.* 2000;24(6):345-350.

[55] Reddy P, Malone M. Cost and outcome analysis of home parenteral and enteral nutrition. *JPEN.* 1998;22(5):302-310.

[56] Howard L, Malone M. Current status of home parenteral nutrition in the United States. *Transplant Proc.* Oct 1996;28(5):2691-2695.

[57] Schalamon J, Mayr JM, Hollwarth ME. Mortality and economics in short bowel syndrome. *Best Pract Res Clin Gastroenterol.* Dec 2003;17(6):931-942.

[58] Sudan D. Cost and Quality of Life After Intestinal Transplantation. *Gastroenterology.* 2006;130:S158–S162.

[59] Olieman JF, Poley MJ, Gischler SJ, et al. Interdisciplinary management of infantile short bowel syndrome: resource consumption, growth, and nutrition. *Journal of Pediatric Surgery.* Mar 2010;45(3):490-498.

[60] DiBaise JK, Scolapio JS. Home parenteral and enteral nutrition. *Gastroenterol Clin North Am.* Mar 2007;36(1):123-144, vii.

[61] Spencer A, Kovacevich D, McKinney-Barnett M, et al. Pediatric short bowel syndrome: The cost of comprehensive care. *Amer J Clin Nutr.* 2008;88:1552-1559.

[62] Jeppesen PB, Pertkiewicz M, Messing B, et al. Teduglutide reduces need for parenteral support among patients with short bowel syndrome with intestinal failure. *Gastroenterology.* Dec 2012;143(6):1473-1481 e1473.

[63] Compher C, Gilroy R, Pertkiewicz M, et al. Maintenance of parenteral nutrition volume reduction, without weight loss, after stopping teduglutide in a subset of patients with short bowel syndrome. *JPEN J Parenter Enteral Nutr.* Sep 2011;35(5):603-609.

In: Short Bowel Syndrome in Children
Editor: Igor Sukhotnik
ISBN: 978-1-62948-518-8

Chapter III

Short Bowel Syndrome: Pathophysiology and Intestinal Adaptation

I. Sukhotnik, M.D.
Department of Pediatric Surgery, Bnai Zion Medical Center,
Laboratory of Intestinal Adaptation and Recovery,
Technion-Israel Institute of Technology,
The Ruth & Bruce Rappaport Faculty of Medicine, Haifa, Israel

Abstract

The degree and extent of malabsorption and metabolic complications seen in short bowel syndrome (SBS) depends on the site of intestinal resection. When the jejunum is resected, a temporary reduction in absorption of most nutrients occurs. However, when a significant portion of jejunum is lost, intestinal adaptation of the ileum can compensate for many of the jejunal functions. Major ileal resections can reduce absorption of fluid, electrolytes, bile acids, and vitamin B12. These functions cannot be taken over by the remaining jejunum. A number of mechanisms contribute to malabsorption after massive resection, including acid hypersecretion, hypergastrinemia, rapid intestinal transit, impaired residual bowel, loss of surface area, bacterial overgrowth in dilated segments of small bowel, and bile acid depletion. Diarrhea in patients with short bowel syndrome is due to a combination of increased secretions, increased motility, and osmotic stimulation of water secretion because of malabsorption of luminal contents. The combined loss of absorptive surface area and compromised enterohepatic circulation, decreased bile acid pool and decreased pancreatic lipase secretion results in steatorrhea and inefficient fat absorption.

Keywords: Short bowel syndrome, physiology, gastrointestinal, nutrient, absorption, malabsorption, malnutrition, diarrhea, steatorrhea, vitamin malabsorption, hypergastrinemia, renal stones, bacterial overgrowth

I. Normal Gastrointestinal Physiology

A basic review of normal gastrointestinal anatomy and physiology is essential to an understanding of the impact of intestinal resection on the clinical outcome and management of patients with short bowel syndrome (SBS). The small intestine is the longest section of the digestive tube and consists of three segments forming a passage from the pylorus to the large intestine: duodenum, jejunum and ileum [1,2]. Nutrient absorption mostly takes place in the jejunum and ileum. The mucosa of these sections is highly folded (the folds are called plicae), increasing the surface area available for absorption dramatically. The jejunum has longer villi and a large absorptive surface area, it has a high concentration of digestive enzymes as well as enzyme carrier proteins and is the site of greatest nutrient absorption including carbohydrate, protein, fat, as well as minerals. The tight junctions are relatively large, rendering the epithelium more porous to larger molecules and the free and rapid flux of water and electrolytes. Villi become shorter and less abundant in the ileum, which therefore has less absorptive surface area than the jejunum. Furthermore, the tight junctions in ileum are tighter, permitting less flux of water and electrolytes from the vascular space into the intestinal lumen, and, consequently, the ileum is more efficient in the absorption of water. Although nutrients are less well absorbed in the ileum, it has site-specific receptors for the absorption of bile acids and vitamin B12. In the term neonate, the small bowel is estimated to be 240 cm, while the colon is about 40 cm [3]. In adult, the normal small intestine varies in length from 365 to 600 cm and has a surface area of 3,300 cm^2 [4]. However, when we include the Kerckring's folds (the numerous circular folds of the mucous membrane, also known as plicae circulares or valvulae conniventes) and the villi and microvilli, the true absorptive surface area are about 2 million cm^2, comparable to the size of a tennis court. Small bowel motility is 3 times slower in the ileum than in the jejunum [5]. The center of each villus is occupied by a capillary network that absorbs nutrients which are eventually transported to the liver by the portal venous system. The terminal ileum has a high concentration of lymphoid tissue that assists in immune regulation. The terminal ileum also has site-specific receptors for absorption of bile acids and vitamin B12. The ileocecal valve plays an important role as a physiologic barrier to the emptying of small bowel into the colon, thus prolonging transit time, and in preventing colonic bacteria from migrating into and contaminating the small bowel. The large intestine, in contrast, is about 150 cm long in most people and does not have villi or a markedly increased absorptive surface. Colonic absorption reduces fluid and electrolyte losses.

Under normal circumstance, newly formed immature intestinal cells divide in the crypts of Lieberkuhn (finger-like invaginations of the epithelium into the underlying connective tissue) and migrate up to the villus tip, differentiate, mature and become functional, with an important role in absorption of nutrients. The renewal process operates continually, with cells taking two to seven days to make the journey from the site of their final division cycle in the crypt to the point of their exfoliation from the villus tip [6]. Intestinal stem cells reside near the base of the crypt, providing immature progeny, which continue to divide as they migrate up the crypt until they differentiate into either intestinal absorptive cells (enterocytes) or secretory lineages (goblet, Paneth, and enteroendocrine cells). Absorptive enterocytes, the primary cell type of the epithelial layer, comprise about 90% of the cells in the entire epithelium and are responsible for the terminal digestion and absorption of luminal nutrients. These cells synthesize digestive enzymes called brush border enzymes that become embedded in the plasma membranes around the microvilli. The goblet cells, located throughout the epithelial layer, secrete mucus that helps protect the epithelial layer from digestion, as well as trefoil factor-3, which is ultimately involved in post-injury repair of the small bowel [7]. The enteroendocrine cells comprise only 1% of the intestinal epithelium and are a part of the enteric endocrine system sense the luminal environment and secrete hormones such as cholecystokinin and gastrin into blood. The overall percentage of secretory lineages within the intestinal epithelium gradually increases from proximal to distal, with the greatest percentage being found in the terminal ileum. The Paneth cells reside at the base of the crypt and are classically believed to have an antimicrobial function in the small intestine (production of lysozyme, an enzyme that destroys bacteria) [8]. The adjacent location of these cells to the intestinal stem cell zone and recent research demonstrating their secretion of cytokines, growth factors, and other products, including soluble WNT proteins known to regulate proliferation, raises the possibility of a potential role for Paneth cells initiating and maintaining the adaptive response [9].

Intestinal growth, gut cell proliferation, cell differentiation, and cell death via apoptosis after massive bowel resection are regulated by reciprocal interactions between the epithelium and the underlying mesenchymal stroma [10]. The formation of intestinal villi is normally preceded by the condensation of mesenchymal cells adjacent to the epithelium at the presumptive sites of new villus formation. As cells begin to differentiate, they migrate towards the lumen and are eventually shed, either from the tips of the intestinal villi or from the surface of the intestinal epithelium. Various signaling cascades have been implicated in the control of stem cell activity, proliferation, lineage commitment, terminal differentiation, and cell survival during normal development and tissue regeneration of the gastrointestinal epithelium. These include Wnt/β-catenin, Hedgehog, bone morphogenetic protein (BMP) and Notch signaling pathways [11-13].

In healthy humans, absorption of fluids and nutrients occurs throughout the length of the small bowel, although to a greater degree in the proximal small bowel, influenced by both concentration and osmotic gradients. In general, virtually all digestion and absorption is completed within the first 100-150 cm of jejunum in a healthy individual. Carbohydrates, proteins, nucleic acids, water and various electrolytes (ions), including Na^+, K^+, Cl^-, nitrates, calcium, and iron are absorbed primarily by facilitated diffusion or active transport in the proximal small bowel. The jejunum is characterized by the relatively porous epithelium. The tight junctions between the epithelial cells, through which many small molecules are transported by solvent drag, have greater diameter in the proximal small intestine [14-15]. The transport of sodium creates an electrochemical gradient and also drives the uptake of carbohydrates and amino acids across the intestinal mucosa. In addition, in the ileum, there is neutral sodium chloride absorption. Water absorption is a passive process resulting from the active transport of nutrients and electrolytes. It has been estimated that the efficiency of water absorption is 44% and 70% of the ingested load in the jejunum and ileum, respectively. For sodium, the corresponding estimates are 13% and 72%, respectively [16]. Hence, the ileum is important in the conservation of fluid and electrolytes. In contrast to the jejunum, the ileum has tighter intercellular junctions resulting in decreased porosity. This leads to less flux of water and sodium and, combined with active transport of sodium chloride in the ileum and colon, allows for significant fluid reabsorption and the ability to concentrate its contents. Lipids and fat-soluble vitamins are packaged and delivered to cells within water-soluble clusters of bile salts called micelles. They are then absorbed by simple diffusion and, once inside the cells, mix with cholesterol and protein to form chylomicrons.

Most of the fats and fat-soluble vitamins are absorbed also in the proximal intestine. The distal small bowel has a primarily role in the absorption of vitamin B12, which combines with intrinsic factor (produced in the stomach) and is absorbed by receptor-mediated endocytosis, and in the active transport of conjugated bile salts. In addition, the ileum acts as a functional reserve for substances not absorbed more proximally. The colon has the slowest transit, varying between 24 and 150 hours.

The intercellular junctions are the tightest in this part of the bowel and the efficiency of water and salt absorption in the colon exceeds 90%. Therefore, patients with the colon in continuity are less likely to suffer from water and electrolyte depletion, particularly as there is a large functional reserve in the colon. Additionally, carbohydrate is fermented in the colon to short-chain fatty acids, which in turn enhance salt and water absorption [17].

II. Pathogenesis of Short Bowel Syndrome

Correlation of Nutrient Malabsorption and Site of Resection

The symptoms associated with SBS are highly dependent upon the site of intestinal resection. Gastrointestinal function in patients with short bowel syndrome is dependent on the anastomotic site and the amount of the remaining intestine. The amount of small bowel remaining after a significant resection is obviously of prime importance in determining how much absorbing surface can participate in the process of nutrient transport. Consequences include malabsorption of fluid, electrolytes, macronutrients, and micronutrients (vitamins and trace elements). A summary of possible consequences of loss of specific intestinal segments is summarized in Table 1.

Table 1. Correlation of nutrient malabsorption and site of resection

Resection of jejunum	Resection of ileum	Resection of ileocecal valve
• Loss of enteric hormone production • Fat malabsorption • Fat-soluble vitamins malabsorption • Calcium malabsorption • Folate malabsorption • Gastric hypersecretion	• Vitamin B12 malabsorption • Bile acid malabsorption • Fat malabsorption	• Increased fluid and electrolyte losses • Bacterial overgrowth

Jejunal resection is not as common as more distal bowel resections and is often necessary for patients with ischemic bowel. In general, jejunal resection is better tolerated than is loss of ileal segments. The jejunum, with its long villi, large absorptive surface, highly concentrated digestive enzymes as well as enzyme carrier proteins, is the primary digestive and absorptive site for most nutrients. The duodenum and jejunum are the primary sites for carbohydrates, proteins, fats, as well as mineral absorption. Thus, when the jejunum is resected, a temporary reduction in absorption of most nutrients occurs. However, when a significant portion of jejunum is lost, intestinal adaptation of the ileum can compensate for many of the jejunal functions. Certain jejunal functions, however, cannot be replaced, including loss of enteric hormone production (such as cholecystokinin and motilin) that affects intestinal motility and digestion. Loss of the jejunum is often accompanied by decreasing biliary and pancreatic secretions and increased gastrin levels, leading to gastric hypersecretion. The remained ileum is characterized by shorter villi, more lymphoid tissue, and a less porous epithelium (compared to resected jejunum) that is less subject to massive fluid losses caused by hypertonic feedings. Therefore, patients in this category can be fed orally immediately and rarely have any problems [18]. However, disease in the ileum and colon may cause the same loss of function as a resection of these segments of the bowel. Ileal resection (with intact jejunum) is commonly performed to manage ileocecal Crohn's disease or necrotizing enterocolitis. The ileum normally reabsorbs a large portion of the fluid secreted by the jejunum during the digestive process, particularly in response to hypertonic feedings [19,20]. If a substantial part of the ileum is resected, fluid and electrolyte loss will occur. Such patients often cannot tolerate large bolus feedings or feedings containing high concentrations of rapidly digested foods (ie, simple carbohydrates). Although the ileum is limited in its capacity to form chylomicrons compared to the jejunum, studies have shown that the ileum has greater adaptive function as far as improving its absorptive function in the presence of short bowel syndrome. Similarly, studies in animals have shown that intestinal transit time is more likely to improve (i.e, increase) in patients with proximal small-bowel resection as opposed to patients with distal small-bowel resection. After an ileal resection, adequate energy and fluid absorption can usually be maintained in the proximal small bowel and colon. However, the distal 100 cm of ileum is the only region that absorbs vitamin B12 and bile salts. While the ileum can adapt and compensate for jejunal loss, the duodenum and jejunum cannot take on the absorptive functions of the ileum. Therefore, major ileal resections can reduce absorption of fluid, electrolytes, bile acids, and vitamin B12. These functions cannot be taken over by the remaining jejunum. In adults, vitamin B12 malabsorption tends to occur if more than 60 cm of ileum is resected, while resection of >100 cm leads to disruption of the enterohepatic circulation, resulting in bile salt deficiency and fat malabsorption [21]. The length of ileal resection that causes such consequences in infants is not well defined. Bile acids, excreted into the duodenum by the liver, are required for the absorption of long-chain fatty acids and fat-soluble vitamins in the ileum. Loss of bile acids may therefore contribute to diarrhea by worsening fat malabsorption. Unabsorbed lipids reaching the ileum cause delay in gastric emptying (the "ileal brake"), which is beneficial because it facilitates absorption of nutrients within the small intestine, and is mediated by hormones secreted by the ileum including peptide YY [22,23]. Ileal resection may be associated with loss of this compensatory mechanism, which may contribute to the diarrhea observed in SBS. The ileocecal valve plays an important role in slowing intestinal transit to allow more time for absorption. The absence of the ileocecal valve, in addition to reducing transit time, can also lead to small bowel bacterial overgrowth colonization by colonic bacteria that can result in mucosal injury and worsening diarrhea. Loss of the ileocecal valve is generally considered to be an important negative predictor of the ability to wean a patient from parenteral nutrition. Absence of the ileocecal valve typically is associated with a longer duration of parenteral nutrition when resection occurs in childhood, and infants with less than 30 cm of small bowel and lacking the ileocecal valve are less likely to be weaned from parenteral nutrition [24,25]. However, another study suggests that the ileocecal valve does not independently affect small bowel transit, the risk of bacterial overgrowth, or the likelihood of weaning from PN [26]. Instead, small bacterial overgrowth was related to small intestinal length and the presence of ileal peristalsis, and these factors were the primary predictors of the likelihood of weaning from parenteral nutrition, rather than the ileocecal valve itself. The colon, if present, can play an important role in absorbing water, sodium, and short-chain fatty acids in SBS patients. The colon also helps to slow intestinal transit and stimulate intestinal adaptation. Loss of the colon in combination with extensive small bowel resection is poorly tolerated and is likely to lead to dehydration and electrolyte depletion. Such patients usually require long-term parenteral nutrition. Moreover, the colon can absorb up to 15 percent of energy requirements, primarily in the form of fermented carbohydrates; in patients with SBS on a high-carbohydrate diet the colon can absorb as much as 50 percent of energy requirements [27,28].

Patients who retain their colon are more likely to tolerate small intestinal resection. As an example, adult patients with SBS but at least half of the colon are likely to have similar intestinal function to those with about 50 cm longer small intestine but no colon [29]. In general, studies in infants and children have reached inconsistent conclusions about whether or not the presence of the colon is an important predictor of weaning from PN [30,31]. By contrast, adults with little or no colon and less than 50 to 100 cm of jejunum are likely to require permanent parenteral nutrition [32]. Thus, the retained colon may be a less important predictor of survival off of PN in infants with SBS as compared with adults.

Decreased production of the bile acid pool causes fat malabsorption with subsequent steatorrhea. Increased diarrhea occurs when colonic bacteria hydroxylate long-chain fatty acids within the colon. Lactose from milk and other liquids is not as easily digested in patients with short bowel syndrome, leading to hyperosmolarity in the intestinal lumen [33]. Furthermore, this malabsorbed lactose in the small intestine becomes fermented in the colon to short chain fatty acids and gases such as hydrogen and carbon dioxide (and in some cases, methane) that produce abdominal discomfort, flatulence, and osmotic diarrhea [34].

III. Mechanisms of Malabsorption

The major effects of massive small bowel resection are summarized in Figure 1.

A number of mechanisms contribute to malabsorption after massive resection, including acid hypersecretion, hypergastrinemia, rapid intestinal transit (especially likely when the distal ileum is resected, or parts of the colon containing peptide YY - the so-called "breaking hormone"- are lost), impaired residual bowel, loss of surface area, bacterial overgrowth in dilated segments of small bowel, and bile acid depletion. Gastric hypersecretion has been attributed to hypergastrinemia following the loss of gastric peptide production from the resected small intestine [35] and can be transient, or may lead to peptic ulcer disease and esophagitis.

Gastric acid hypersecretion is a common finding after massive small bowel resection and is proportional to the length of intestine resected. The increased gastric secretions and acidity inactivate pancreatic enzymes, reducing the efficiency of protein and lipid digestion [36]. The excess gastric acid and low intraduodenal pH may damage the bowel mucosa, inactivate digestive enzymes, and stimulate peristalsis [37]. As a result, many patients benefit from acid suppression using histamine 2 receptor antagonists or a proton pump inhibitor, particularly during the early phase of SBS.

Diarrhea in patient with short bowel syndrome is due to a combination of increased secretions, increased motility, and osmotic stimulation of water secretion because of malabsorption of luminal contents. Hypertonic concentration of partially digested nutrients in the jejunum results in massive fluid losses that would normally be reabsorbed in the ileum and colon. If the ileum is resected, one of the primary reabsorptive sites for these secretions is lost, and the remaining colon is incapable of reabsorbing most of the fluid. Consequently, patient with distal bowel resection usually develop massive fluid losses in response to large bolus feeding, or feedings containing high concentrations of rapidly digested carbohydrates [38].

Carbohydrates in the diet are a major cause of diarrhea in SBS because of their high osmotic load. This is especially true with simple carbohydrates that are osmotically active. Even complex carbohydrates may be a problem because they can create a significant osmotic load in the small bowel after digestion by pancreatic enzymes. In the colon, further breakdown of these compounds by gut bacteria creates additional osmotic loads and fluid losses [39].

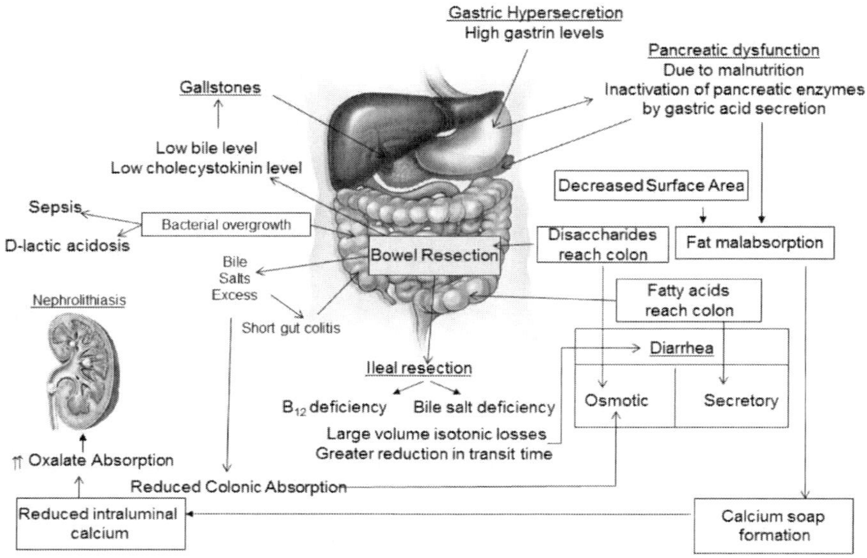

Figure 1. The major effects of massive small bowel resection.

Protein in the diet is usually well-tolerated as a calorie source, and contributes relatively little to the osmotic load, probably because it is not present in large quantities. Fats are large molecules and do not create an osmotic load in the small intestine.

Because they also are a dense source of calories relative to carbohydrates and proteins, they are a valuable source of calories in patients with SBS [40]. The degree of malabsorption increases with the length of resection, and the variety of nutrients malabsorbed increases [41]. Balance studies of energy absorption showed that the absorption of fat and carbohydrate was equally reduced to between 50% and 75% of intake [42]. However, nitrogen absorption was reduced to a lesser extent than that of carbohydrate and fat, namely to 81% of intake. Although the ability to absorb many nutrients is decreased following resection, lipid absorption is generally considered the most vulnerable [43,44]. The combined loss of absorptive surface area and compromised enterohepatic circulation [45] decreased bile acid pool [46] and decreased pancreatic lipase secretion [47] resulting in steatorrhea and inefficient fat absorption. Fats are relatively large molecules that exit the small intestine into the colon without exerting a significant osmotic load and, consequently, do not significantly contribute to osmotic diarrhea. However, fatty acids may stimulate colonic water secretion. Therefore, patients with short bowel syndrome have been considered to benefit from a low-fat diet early in the course of therapy [48].

A review of the literature prior to the availability of parenteral nutrition shows that resections up to 33% result in no malnutrition, and those up to 50% could be tolerated without special aids, but those in excess of 75% require nutritional support to avoid severe malnutrition [49]. Absorption of calcium, magnesium, zinc, and phosphorus is reduced in SBS patient, but does not correlate with the remaining length of the bowel [50]. In addition to malabsorption, diarrhea results in excessive losses of zinc and selenium but not copper [51].

The potential nutrient absorptive function of the colon following small bowel resection has not been fully evaluated. However, the colon does have the capacity to "salvage" malabsorbed carbohydrate by absorbing the short-chain fatty acids resulting from colonic fermentation [52]. Colonic bacteria deconjugate the bile salts entering the colon to free bile acids that stimulate secretion, leading to the development of watery diarrhea. Therefore, the severity of diarrhea following ileal resection depends in part on the length of contiguous colon removed [53].

The gastrointestinal tract is also the site of synthesis of a number of important gastrointestinal hormones and growth factors. Many of these play an important role in regulating gastric emptying and small intestinal transit. Resection of the ileum results in delayed gastric emptying that is a major factor in adaptive increased transit time [54].

On the other hand, resection of the ileum may impair the "colon brake" phenomenon thought to be controlled by neurotensin and peptide YY [55]. Consequently, the presence of malabsorptive fat in the distal ileum will not have its usual ability to reduce intestinal motility, and permit greater contact of nutrients with the epithelial surface to aid absorption [51]. Low peptide YY values in patients with short bowel without a colon may be partly responsible for the high volume of jejunostomy output. Other compounds, including prostaglandins, cholecystokinin, and secretin, were not found to adequately maintain the mucosa in the setting of TPN [57]. Decreased secretion of cholecystokinin and secretin further reduces gallbladder contraction and pancreatic secretion. These factors along with secretion of a high salt load by the stomach may compound the diarrhea associated with short bowel syndrome [58].

IV. Intestinal Adaptation

A. Definition of Adaptation

Although intestinal transplantation has emerged as a feasible alternative in the treatment of children with short bowel syndrome (SBS) during the last two decades, intestinal adaptation remains the only chance for survival in a subset of these patients. Intestinal adaptation may be defined as a progressive recovery from intestinal failure throughout which the small bowel increases its absorptive surface area and its functional capacity in an attempt to increase fluid and nutrient absorption and to meet the body's metabolic and growth needs [59]. In the early twentieth century it was first observed that massive small bowel resection led to "compensatory hypertrophy" of the remaining gut [60]. In 1957 Pilling and Cresson [61] described the first successful extensive resection in two infants, who survived with only 26 and 28 cm of remaining small bowel. Subsequently, many series of patients have demonstrated survival in infants with even shorter small bowel remnants [62,63].

In humans, intestinal adaptation begins within 24-48 hours of resection and includes morphologic (structural adaptation) and functional changes (functional adaptation) of the residual bowel. Structural adaptation includes increasing bowel diameter and length, lengthening the villi, deepening the crypts, and increasing the rate of enterocyte proliferation, finally resulting in increased absorptive surface area and in increased numbers of enterocytes. Functional adaptation entails modifications of the brush border membrane permeability and up-regulation of carrier-mediated transport, ultimately resulting in increased nutrient absorption by isolated enterocytes [60,61]. Several studies have shown that the functional integrity of the remaining intestine is of far more importance than the outward appearance of the bowel [64]. The nutritional benefits of an increased intestinal absorption in short bowel patients are usually reflected in changes of body weight and composition. The increases in the body weight and lean body and bone mass, and the reduction in the fat mass seen as a result of the conservative treatment may be taken as clinical indications of a beneficial effect, which most probably is mediated through the effect on intestinal absorption. In addition, the increase in urine creatinine and the absence of clinical signs of edema supported that the increase in lean body mass, measured by dual-energy x-ray absorptiometry, actually reflect an increase in muscle mass. The increases in serum albumin and sodium are also encouraging [65]. Figure 1 illustrates a theoretic graphic presentation of gut function in relation to time after bowel resection. A "Spontaneous adaptation," or recovery of intestinal function is generally described, reaching a plateau at a certain time (usually after 18 months). When trying to improve intestinal adaptation, therapies could either reach a higher plateau phase (given as graph "Enhanced adaptation"), or reduce the time period until the plateau was reached (given as graph "Accelerated adaptation"). Enhanced accelerated adaptation refers to situation when adaptation reaches higher plateau and in shorter time. Accelerating the process may be relevant in patients who are difficult to maintain on parenteral nutrition. However, the maximal increase in the functional absorptive capacity obtained by enhanced adaptation, represented by the level of the plateau, is the aim when trying to wean stable patients from parenteral support.

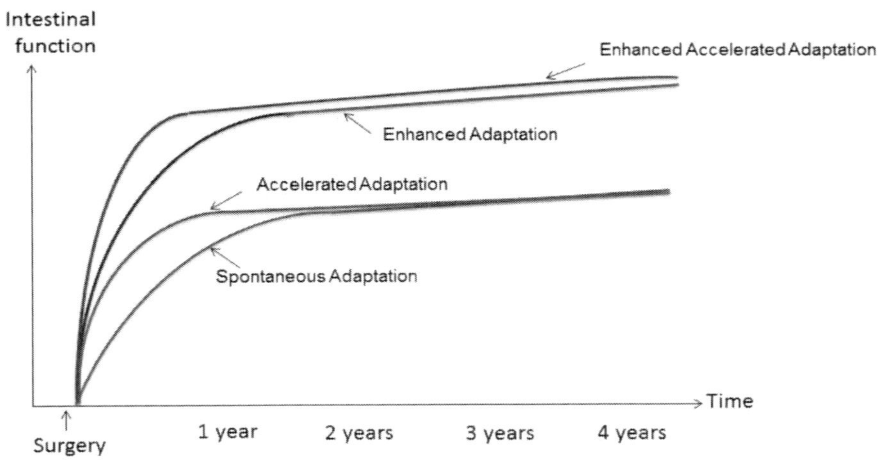

Figure 2. Theoretic graphic presentation of gut function during intestinal adaptation.

B. Mechanisms of Adaptation

Most studies investigating the process of adaptation have utilized animal models (rat, mouse and dog) with a jejunoileal anastomosis. Therefore, the relevance of the physiological and structural changes that occur is of unclear clinical relevance to humans who uncommonly have this bowel anatomy remaining. Hyperplasia of the mucosal epithelium, not hypertrophy, is the primary event occurring in intestinal adaptation [66,67]. In rodent systems, animals subjected to extensive (70%) intestinal resection undergo a pattern of well described morphological and functional changes. The remaining intestine changes macroscopically with dilatation, thickening, and an increasing length. There is an increase in villus height and diameter, and an elongation of the crypts. Increased villus height and crypt depth are the result of increased proliferation and accelerated migration along the villus, and is a marker for the increased absorptive surface area. Increased mucosal proliferation in a functioning intestine, as demonstrated by the increased cell proliferation index following bowel resection, suggests an activated enterocyte turnover and may be considered as a main mechanism of mucosal hyperplasia in residual bowel. An increase in epithelial cellular proliferation, coupled with an increase in apoptosis, produces increases in intestinal RNA, DNA, and protein content [68,69]. The dynamic process of enterocyte turnover is a function of the rates of crypt cell proliferation, migration along crypt-villus axis, and death via apoptosis. This process may be affected by nutritional status, the route of feeding, and the adequacy of specific nutrients in the diet. Apoptosis, or programmed cell death is an active, genetically controlled process of cell suicide. It is a physiologic process whereby the body disposes of unwanted cells by self-destruction and is our greatest defense against damaged cells [70]. In contrast to necrosis, which is more of an accidental death process, apoptosis comprises highly regulated and reproducible events that eventually lead to cell death. Several regulatory genes affecting apoptosis have been identified and divided into pro-apoptotic genes (bax, bik, bak, bcl-xs, bad, p53, c-jun, hrk) and anti-apoptotic genes (bcl-2, bcl-x_L, rb, mcl-1, a1, brag-1, bfl-1) [71]. Many reports on apoptosis focused on the role of the executioners, **C**ysteinyl-**asp**arate-acid-protein**ases,** termed "caspases" which are triggered in response to pro-apoptotic signals. Caspases cleave numerous substrates at the carboxyl side of an aspirate residue upon induction of apoptosis. A key caspase involved in the apoptotic pathway is caspase-3 (also known as Yama, CPP32, and Apopain). Inhibition of caspase-3 has been linked to prevention of apoptotic death in-vitro, although certain stimuli can induce apoptosis by a caspase-3-independent pathway [72]. Bcl-2 and related proteins play an important role in the regulation of apoptotic cell death in mammalian systems [73]. At least two family members, Bcl-xs and Bax, act in opposition to Bcl-2. Recent evidence has demonstrated that apoptosis increases in SBS [74]. Enhanced enterocyte apoptosis following bowel resection is considered as being a mechanism that counterbalances the increased enterocyte proliferation in order to reach a new homeostatic status during intestinal adaptation, promoting the disposal of genetically aberrant stem cells and preventing tumorigenesis. In a recent experiment, Jarboe et al. [75] examined the role of *bax* in exaggerated post-resection apoptosis induced by epidermal growth factor receptor inhibition in mice and demonstrated that *bax* is required for the induction of such cell death. Moreover, defective epidermal growth factor receptor signaling augmented resection-induced enterocyte apoptosis via a mechanism that also requires *bax* expression. Functionally there is an increase in absorption per unit length of carbohydrates, proteins, water, and electrolytes [76,77]. In response to a variety of stimuli, including luminal nutrients, hormones, growth factors, and pancreaticobiliary secretions, the small and large intestine increase their absorptive surface area and functional capacity to meet the body's metabolic and growth needs.

C. Enhancing Adaptation

Considerable research over many years has focused on the identification of those trophic factors that may promote bowel absorption after massive intestinal resection and provide a successful outcome in patients with SBS. These factors include nutrients and other luminal constituents, gastrointestinal secretions, hormones and peptide growth factors [78-80].

Adaptation and Nutrients

It is well documented that exposure to intraluminal nutrients is required for stimulation of intestinal adaptation in general and mucosal hyperplasia in particular [78]. Therefore, many experts in the management of SBS recommend attempting enteral feeding as early as possible. The mechanism whereby food induces this adaptation is unknown. It is likely that enteral nutrition works through a number of mechanisms, including stimulation of mucosal hyperplasia by direct contact with the epithelial cells, stimulation of trophic gastrointestinal hormone secretion and stimulation of the production of trophic pancreaticobiliary secretions [65,66]. Although enteral feeding is one of the major trophic factors in the stimulation of intestinal adaptation, not all nutrients have equal stimulating trophic effects. Growing evidence suggest that glutamine, pectin, short chain fatty acids and long chain fatty acids are considered the most effective among the factors promoting post-resection intestinal adaptation [65]. The main mechanism of lipid absorption is by passive diffusion, although the evidence for protein facilitated transfer is accumulating. Fatty acid binding protein (FABP) and fatty acid translocase (FAT/CD36) are expressed in the intestine and upregulated after resection in rodents [79,80]. However, this is not accompanied by the increased intestinal uptake of long chain fatty acids [81]. Essential fatty acids may be required for optimal adaptation after resection. Rats fed fatty acid deficient diets had reduced mucosal hyperplasia compared with controls [82]. However, a low fat normo-caloric diet reduces, but does not abolish the adaptive response. Although lipid absorption is generally considered the most vulnerable in SBS patient, growing evidence suggests that long chain fatty acids appear to be more effective stimulators of intestinal adaptation than either medium-chain fats or carbohydrates [83]. Early exposure to a high fat diet augmented and accelerated intestinal re-growth after massive small bowel resection in a rat model [84]. In addition, dietary lipids increased the absorptive capacity of the intestinal remnant, improved food and fat absorption, and restored plasma and tissue lipid content in this model [85,86]. In contrast, a low fat diet significantly affected adaptive responses by an inhibition of enterocyte proliferation and did so independently of enterocyte apoptosis [87]. Depletion of dietary fat also inhibited cellular and molecular mechanisms of LCFA absorption by isolated enterocytes in the same model. This was evident from a decrease in LCFA plasma-membrane transport protein fatty-acid translocase (FAT) (the rat homologue of human CD36), and a decrease in isolated enterocyte [3H]-oleate uptake as measured by established cellular LCFA transport assay [88].

Extensive studies in various experimental models of SBS have established that many amino acids (for example, glutamine) strongly stimulate the intestinal adaptive response. Glutamine, rather than glucose, is the major fuel for mitochondrial respiration in enterocytes. Glutamine is used for protein synthesis either directly or as a result of catabolic pathways. Within 24 hours of 80% small bowel resection in the rodent, glutamine and total amino acid uptake per gram of tissue is increased [89]. However, with the decrease mass of tissue, overall glutamine consumption in the long term is less than controls and muscle stores of glutamine remain unchanged [90-92]. The addition of glutamine or arginine to enteral feeds after extensive resection does not seem to produce a consistent effect between studies; indeed, there is little evidence that either amino acid increases adaptation, with some groups reporting lower protein and DNA levels than controls [93]. Supplementation of enteral feeds with ornithine a ketoglutarate (OKG), the soluble ornithine salt, does seem to have a positive effect on intestinal adaptation and mucosal polyamine synthesis [94]. Vitamin A is essential for normal growth and for differentiation of epithelial tissues. Extensive studies in various experimental models have established that vitamin A may regulate intestinal epithelial cell proliferation and regeneration [95].

Intestinal Adaptation and Hormones

It is widely accepted that the adaptive response is controlled in part by the release of one or more of the gut signaling hormones. These include enteroglucagon, neurotensin, peptide YY, growth hormone, and insulin like growth factor [96]. Enteroendocrine glucagon-like peptides GLP-1 and GLP-2 are synthesized and released from enteroendocrine cells in the distal small intestine and large intestine. GLP-1 promotes efficient nutrient assimilation while GLP-2 regulates energy absorption via effects on nutrient intake, gastric acid secretion and gastric emptying, nutrient absorption, and mucosal permeability [97]. Growing evidence suggests that GLP-2 is important in controlling intestinal adaptation following bowel resection [98-100]. Administration of GLP2 may improve nutrient absorption in patients with no colon. Eight patients, with SBS, all of whom had undergone ileal and colonic resection were given 400 mg of GLP2 subcutaneously, twice daily for five weeks. Improvements with treatment compared with controls were seen in intestinal absorption of energy, wet weight, nitrogen, as well as increases in lean body mass and overall body weight. There were no changes in transit time. There were minimal adverse effects described and patient compliance was good [101]. However, only four patients in this study actually required home TPN.

Recent studies have shown that treatment with bombesin caused increased mitotic activity in crypt cells and improved nutrient absorption after massive small bowel resection in a rat [102]. In another recent study, treatment with bombesin resulted in a significant increase in accelerated cell turnover after massive small bowel resection in a rat [103]. The obese gene protein product leptin is a hormone that is secreted from adipocytes and acts primarily on the hypothalamus regulating energy expenditure and food intake [104-106]. Recent study has shown that treatment with leptin enhances structural intestinal adaptation, increases enterocyte proliferation and decreases cell death via apoptosis following massive small bowel resection in a rat [107].

Because of its antisecretory properties, somatostatin has been advocated for the treatment of patients with SBS. Somatostatin decreases diarrhea and stoma output following massive small bowel resection. However, recent experimental evidence suggests that sandostatin decreases cell proliferation and inhibits structural intestinal adaptation following massive small bowel resection in a rat model [108]. In light of these results, somatostatin should be avoided following massive small bowel resection in order to prevent its inhibitory effects of bowel re-growth.

Little is known about the effects of gender and sex hormones in short bowel syndrome. A growing body of literature points to gender differences in many diseases as well as gender dimorphism in the response to trauma, shock and sepsis. Current theories for the different responses to these events between genders are based on gonadal, hypothalamic and pituitary hormone levels. In a recent study, the effects of gender and sex hormones on structural intestinal adaptation were investigated following massive small bowel resection in a rat [109]. This study confirms that bowel re-growth following massive small bowel resection is not gender related. Depletion of androgen by castration inhibited intestinal adaptation, and testosterone showed a strong stimulating effect on bowel re-growth.

Growth hormone (GH) is a single chain protein produced in the anterior pituitary gland. Because GH has been shown to induce growth and proliferation in many different tissues and cell lines and the receptor for growth hormone has been found throughout the intestine, its role in the setting of SBS has been studied extensively. Many studies in various experimental models of SBS have established that exogenous administration of growth hormone enhances mucosal hyperplasia and increases water, electrolytes and nutrient absorption [110,111]. Treated animals have shown mucosal hyperplasia and increased absorptive capacity above and beyond the normal adaptive response after small bowel resection. Other studies have demonstrated increased villus height and crypt depth, positive nitrogen balance and bowel growth when rats were given GH combined with glutamine and/or a diet high in protein [112,113]. These studies do not discredit GH as a driver of adaptation but underscores the interplay between the many factors involved in adaptation in SBS. Another very promising observation is that GH may augment the length of the remnant intestine after bowel resection. This finding is particularly important when you consider that remnant intestinal length is the greatest predictor for long term parenteral nutrition requirement.

Adaptation and Peptide Growth Factors

Over the past decades several proteins produced by different cells and tissues, designated peptide growth factors, have been reported to play an important role in stimulating enterocyte turnover. Peptide growth factors appear to mediate many of the processes required for normal intestinal growth and differentiation. Every growth factor modulates growth through autocrine, juxtacrine or paracrine mechanisms and usually acts as a mitogen through the stimulation of specific cell surface receptors. It has been reported that growth factors stimulate cell proliferation through the alteration of transcription of various genes. Peptide growth factors are often divided into several groups based on their structure and mode of induction, and include the epidermal growth factor (EGF) family, the transforming growth factor β (TGFβ) family, the insulin like growth factor (IGF) family, and the fibroblast growth factor (FGF) family. In addition, a smaller number of peptide growth factors having different structural properties compared to the main families also have been identified within the gastrointestinal tract. These include hepatocyte growth factor (HGF), platelet derived growth factor (PDGF), trefoil peptides, hematopoietic stem cell factors and many more.

Certain peptide growth factors have been evaluated for their role in modifying cell proliferation and in stimulating the enterocyte functional activities in animal models of short bowel syndrome. The effect of other factors has not been evaluated following bowel resection and further work is required to study their effect on intestinal adaptation. The Epidermal growth factor (EGF) family includes epidermal growth factor, transforming growth factor-alpha (TGF-α), and heparin binding epidermal-like growth factor. All bind the EGF receptor (c-erbB-1) that is expressed on the basolateral surface of intestinal epithelial cells. EGF is produced by the Brunner glands of the duodenum and in salivary glands. Epidermal growth factor has been shown to augment the intestinal adaptation in animal models of SBS. Multiple studies have suggested a positive effect of EGF on both structural and functional parameters of intestinal adaptation [114]. The second member of the EGF family, transforming growth factor-α (TGF-α), is a 50-amino-acid polypeptide which was first identified in nontransformed fibroblasts indicator cells in soft agar and was found to promote anchorage-independent growth of these cells. TGF-α shares many structural homologies to EGF and appears to act through the same receptor as EGF. In a recent study, exogenous TGF-α stimulated cell proliferation, inhibited cell apoptosis and enhanced intestinal structural adaptation following massive small bowel resection in a rat [115]. In the other experiment, effects of TGF-α on enterocyte turnover were evaluated in correlation with epidermal-growth factor (EGF) receptor expression along the villus-crypt axis in a rat model of SBS. Villus tips, lateral villi and crypts were separated using laser capture microdissection. EGF receptor expression for each compartment was assessed by quantitative real-time PCR. This study has shown that the effect of TGF-α on enterocyte turnover is correlated with EGF receptor expression along the villus-crypt axis [116]. In every compartment, the increase of EGF receptor expression coincided with increased cell proliferation and decreased cell apoptosis following TGF-α administration (Figure 3).

The insulin-like growth factor family includes three peptides: insulin, insulin-like growth factor I (IGF-I), and insulin-like growth factor II (IGF-II). Growth hormone mediates its trophic effects by IGF-I. IGF-I produces its main biological actions through the type-1 insulin-like growth factor receptor, which is distributed uniformly on epithelial cells through the small intestine, but is present to a higher degree in the colon [117]. In serum, IGF-I is bound to circulating binding proteins (insulin like growth factor binding proteins (IGFBP)). The IGFBPs can also have independent effects on cell growth. The positive effect of IGF-I and IGF-II in stimulating bowel re-growth after intestinal resection has been reported by many investigators [118,119].

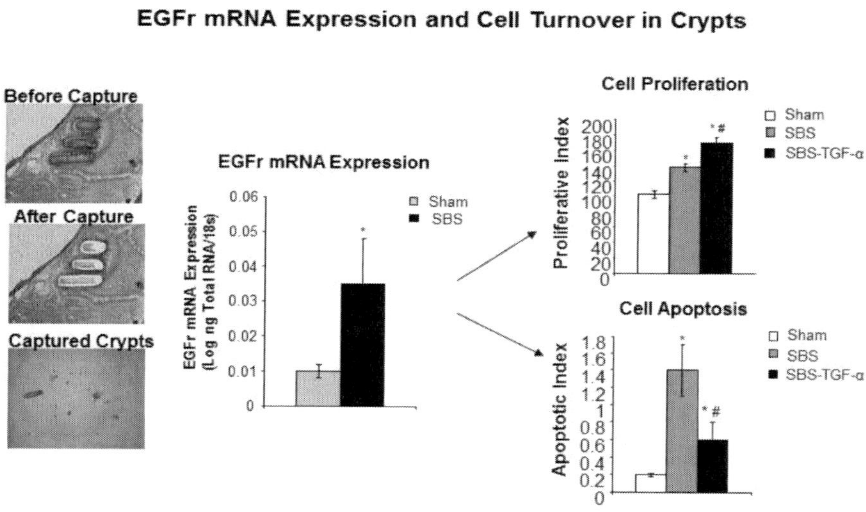

Figure 3. Relationship between EGFr mRNA expression and enterocyte turnover in crypts following massive small bowel resection and treatment with TGF-a SBS- short bowel syndrome rats; EGFr epidermal growth factor receptor, TGF-a transforming growth factor-alpha Values are mean ± SEM. *P<0.05 SBS versus Sham rats, #P<0.05 SBS- TGF-a versus SBS rats (adapted from Sukhotnik at al.).

In a recent study, oral insulin supplementation dramatically enhanced structural intestinal adaptation after massive bowel resection in a rat [120]. This effect was much more significant than the one observed previously following parenteral insulin administration and was correlated with insulin receptor expression along the villus-crypt axis [121]. Based on these studies, a pilot study was performed to examine whether oral insulin supplementation decreases the need for parenteral nutrition in pediatric patients with SBS. In this trial, clinical improvement was observed in a subset of children, with two of ten infants successfully weaned off parenteral nutrition [122]. Fibroblast growth factors play key roles in controlling tissue growth, morphogenesis, and repair in animals. Keratinocyte growth factor (KGF, fibroblast growth factor VII) is produced locally in the gut by intraepithelial lymphocytes and stromal cells in the lamina propria, and induces epithelial cell proliferation and up-regulates antiapoptotic factors in the intestine. A recent study has shown that keratinocyte growth factor plays a positive role in intestinal re-growth in a mouse model of SBS [123]. The transforming growth factor beta (TGF-β) superfamily consists of about 30 structurally related proteins. These include 3 isoforms of TGF-β (TGF-β1-3) itself, 3 forms of activin and over 20 bone morphogenetic proteins (BMPs). TGF-β has been found to bind to several specific cell surface receptors. The type-1 and type-2 receptors work in a cooperative fashion: ligand binding to the type-1 receptor facilitates activation of the associated type-2 receptor, which then activates the intracellular signaling machine via SMAD proteins. TGF-b family plays an important role in regulating cell growth and development [124,125]. In a recent study, the effect of dietary supplementation with TGFβ2 on intestinal adaptation and enterocyte turnover after massive small bowel resection in a rat was investigated. This study has shown that enteral supplementation with TGF-β2 inhibits intestinal adaptation with inhibited enterocyte proliferation being responsible for this effect [126].

Intestinal growth, gut cell proliferation, cell differentiation, and cell death via apoptosis after massive bowel resection are regulated by reciprocal interactions between the epithelium and the underlying mesenchymal stroma. Growing evidence suggests that platelet-derived growth factor (PDGF) signaling is an important mediator of these interactions. The formation of intestinal villi is normally preceded by the condensation of mesenchymal cells adjacent to the epithelium at the presumptive sites of new villus formation. Changes in the stromal environment may indirectly contribute to changes in the number and size of the crypts as well as allow their progressive invasion of villus tissue. A recent experiment has shown that 1) bowel resection in a rat results in activation of PDGF signaling; 2) exogenous PDGF-α stimulates intestinal re-growth after resection; and 3) the stimulating effect of PDGF-α on enterocyte turnover (proliferation and apoptosis) is correlated with PDGF-α receptor expression along the villus-crypt axis [127].

The effects of other growth factors on bowel growth have been examined in normal intestine, but have not been evaluated in an animal model of short bowel syndrome. Future experiments will, therefore, be needed to examine the role of these factors and to elucidate the potential mechanisms by which they affect the adaptive response.

Conflict of Interest

None declared.

Acknowledgment

None declared.

References

[1] Ellis H. Anatomy of the small intestine (jejunum and ileum). *Surgery* (Oxford), 2011; 29:355-7.

[2] Osunkotun B, Kocoshis SA. Anatomy and physiology of the small and large intestine: Wyllie R, Hyams JS, Kay M (eds). *Pediatric Gastrointestinal and Liver Disease*. Elsevier; 2006, Pp 459–474.

[3] Touloukian RJ, Smith GJW. Normal intestinal length in preterm infants. *J Pediatr Surg* 1983; 18: 720-3.

[4] Shatari T, Clark MA, Lee JR, Keighley MR. Reliability of radiographic measurement of small intestinal length. *Colorectal Dis* 2004; 6:327-9.

[5] Summers RW, Kent TH, Osborne JW. Effects of drugs, ileal obstruction and irradiation on rat gastrointestinal propulsion. *Gastroenterology* 1970; 59:731-9.

[6] Wright N, Alison M. *The biology of epithelial cell populations*. Clarendon, Oxford, 1984.

[7] Beck PL, Wong JF, Li Y, Swaminathan S, Xavier RJ, Devaney KL,and Podolsky DK. Chemotherapy- and radiotherapy-induced intestinal damage is regulated by intestinal trefoil factor. *Gastroenterology* 2004; 126:796–808.

[8] Garabedian EM, Roberts LJJ, McNevin MS, Gordon JI. Examining the role of Paneth cells in the small intestine by lineage ablation in transgenic mice. *J Biol Chem* 1997; 272: 23729-40.

[9] Bjerknes M, Cheng H. The stem-cell zone of the small intestinal epithelium. I. Evidence from Paneth cells in the adult mouse. *Am J Anat* 1981; 160: 51–63.

[10] Booth C, Potten CS. Gut instincts: thoughts on intestinal epithelial stem cells. *J Clin Invest* 2000;105:1493-9.

[11] Goumans MJ, Mummery C. Functional analysis of the TGFb receptor/Smad pathway through gene ablation in mice. *Int J Dev Biol* 2000;44: 253-65.

[12] Chiba S. Notch signaling in stem cell systems. *Stem Cells*, 2006; 24:2437-47.

[13] Radtke F, Clevers H. Self-renewal and cancer of the gut: two sides of a coin. *Science* 2005;307: 1904-9.

[14] Pinto D, Clevers H. Wnt control of stem cells and differentiation in the intestinal epithelium. *Exp Cell Res* 2005;306:357-63.

[15] Fordtran JS, Rector JF Jr, Ewton MF, Soter N, Kinney J. Permeability characteristics of the human small inytestine. *J X Clin Invest* 1968:47: 884-900.

[16] Fordtran JS, Locklear TW. Ionic constituent and osmolality of gastric and small intestinal fluids after eating. *Am J Dig Dis* 1966; 11:503-21.

[17] Powell DW. Intestinal water and electrolyte transport. In: Johnson JR, ed. *Physiology of the gastrointestinal tract.* 2nd ed. New York: Raven Press, 1987.

[18] Binder HJ, Mehta P. Short-chain fatty acids stimulate active sodium and chloride absorption in vitro in the rat distal colon. *Gastroenterology* 1989; 96:989-96.

[19] Fordtran JS, Rector FC Jr, Carter NW. The mechanisms of sodium absorption in the human small intestine. *J Clin Invest* 1968; 47:884-886.

[20] Fordtran JS, Rector FC Jr, Ewton MF. Permeability characteristics of the human small intestine. J Clin Invest 1965; 44:1935.Parekh NR, Steiger E. Short bowel syndrome. *Curr Treat Options Gastroenterol* 2007;10:10-23.

[21] Hofmann AF, Poley JR. Role of bile acid malabsorption in pathogenesis of diarrhea and steatorrhea in patients with ileal resection. I. Response to cholestyramine or replacement of dietary long chain triglyceride by medium chain triglyceride. *Gastroenterology* 1972;62:918-923.

[22] Welch IM, Cunningham KM, Read NW. Regulation of gastric emptying by ileal nutrients in humans. *Gastroenterology* 1988; 94:401-5.

[23] Van Citters GW, Lin HC. Ileal brake: neuropeptidergic control of intestinal transit. *Curr Gastroenterol Rep* 2006; 8:367-71.

[24] Goulet OJ, Revillon Y, Jan D, et al. Neonatal short bowel syndrome. *J Pediatr* 1991; 119:18-23.

[25] Goulet O, Baglin-Gobet S, Talbotec C. Outcome and long-term growth after extensive small bowel resection in the neonatal period: a survey of 87 children. *Eur J Pediatr Surg* 2005; 15:95-9.

[26] Kaufman SS, Loseke CA, Lupo JV, Young RJ, Murray ND, Pinch LW, Vanderhoof JA. Influence of bacterial overgrowth and intestinal inflammation on duration of parenteral nutrition in children with short bowel syndrome. *J Pediatr* 1997;131:356-9.

[27] DiBaise JK, Young RJ, Vanderhoof JA. Intestinal rehabilitation and the short bowel syndrome: part 2. *Am J Gastroenterol* 2004; 99:1823-8.

[28] Jeppesen PB, Mortensen PB. Significance of a preserved colon for parenteral energy requirements in patients receiving home parenteral nutrition. *Scand J Gastroenterol* 1998; 33:1175-9.

[29] Nightingale JM, Lennard-Jones JE, Gertner DJ. Colonic preservation reduces need for parenteral therapy, increases incidence of renal stones, but does not change high prevalence of gall stones in patients with a short bowel. *Gut* 1992; 33:1493-9.

[30] Diamond IR, Struijs MC, de Silva NT, Wales PW. Does the colon play a role in intestinal adaptation in infants with short bowel syndrome? A multiple variable analysis. *J Pediatr Surg* 2010; 45:975-80.

[31] Spencer AU, Neaga A, West B. Pediatric short bowel syndrome: redefining predictors of success. *Ann Surg* 2005; 242:403-8.

[32] Gouttebel MC, Saint-Aubert B, Astre C, Joyeux H. Total parenteral nutrition needs in different types of short bowel syndrome. *Dig Dis Sci* 1986; 31:718-24.

[33] Dudrick SJ, Latifi R. Management of short-bowel syndrome. In: Kirby DF, Dudrick SJ, eds. *Practical handbook of nutrition in clinical practice*. Boca Raton: CRC Press, 1994.

[34] Beyer PL, Flynn MA. Effect of high- and low-fiber diets on human feces. *J Am Diet Assoc* 1978; 72:271-2.

[35] Hyman PE, Everett SL, Harada T. Gastric acid hypersecretion in short bowel syndrome in infants: association with extent of resection and enteral feeding. *J Pediatr Gastroenterol Nutr* 1986;5:191-7.

[36] Wright JK. Short gut syndrome- options for management. *Compr Ther* 1992; 18:5–8.

[37] Williams NS, Evans P, King RF. Gastric acid secretion and gastrin production in the short bowel syndrome. *Gut* 1985;26:914-9.

[38] Vanderhoof JA, Langnas AN. Short bowel syndrome in children and adults. *Gastroenterology* 113: 1767-1778, 1997-2003.

[39] Nordgaard I, Hansen BS, Mortensen PB. Colon as a digestive organ in patients with short bowel. *Lancet* 1994;343:373-6.

[40] Bongaerts GP, Severijnen RS. Arguments for a lower carbohydrate-higher fat diet in patients with a short small bowel. *Med Hypotheses* 2006;67:280-5.

[41] Hylander E, Ladefoged K, Jarnum S. Nitrogen absorption following small intestinal resection. *Scand J Gastroenterol* 1980;15:853-8.

[42] Woolf GM, Miller C, Kurian R, Jeejeebhoy KN. Nutritional absorption in short bowel syndrome: evaluation of fluid, calorie, and divalent cation requirements. *Dig Dis Sci* 1987;32:8-15.

[43] Vanderhoof JA, Burkley KT, Antonson KT. Potential for mucosal adaptation following massive small bowel resection in 3-week-old versus 8-week-old rats. *J Pediatr Gastroenterol Nutr* 1983;2:672-6.

[44] Chiba T, Ohi R. Do we still need to collect stool? Evaluation of visualized fatty acid absorption: experimental studies using rats. *J Parenter Enteral Nutr* 1998; 22:22-6.

[45] Molina MT, Ruiz-Cutierrez V, Vazquez CM. Changes in uptake of linoleic acid and cholesterol by jejunal sacs of rats in vitro, after distal small bowel resection. *Scand J Gastroenterol* 1990; 25:613-21.

[46] Tilson MD, Boyer JL, Wright HK. Jejunal absorption of bile salts after resection of the ileum. *Surgery* 1975;77:231-4.

[47] Pitchumoni CS. Pancreas in primary malnutrition disorders. *Am J Clin Nutr* 1973; 26:374-9.

[48] Biller JA. Short bowel syndrome. In: Grand RI, Sutphen JL, Dietz WH (eds) *Pediatric nutrition. Theory and practice.* Butterworth, Stoneham, MA,1987; pp 481–487.

[49] Haymond HE. Massive resection of the small intestine: analysis of 257 collected cases. *Surg Gynecol Obstet* 1953;61:693-705.

[50] Ladefoged K, Nicolaidou P, Jarnum S. Calcium, phosphorus, magnesium, zinc and nitrogen balance in patients with severe short bowel syndrome. *Am J Clin Nutr* 1980;33:2137-44.

[51] Wolman SL, Anderson GH, Marliss EB, Jeejeebhoy KN. Zinc in total parenteral nutrition: requirements and metabolic effects. *Gastroenterology* 1979;76:458-67.
[52] Ruppin H, Bar-Meir S, Soergel KH, Wood CM, Schmitt MG Jr. Absorption of short-chain fatty acids by the colon. *Gastroenterology* 1980; 78:1500-7.
[53] Mitchel JE, Breuer KI, Zuckerman L, Berlin J, Schilli L, Dunn JK. The colon influences ileal resection diarrhea. *Dig Dis Sci* 1980; 25:33-41.
[54] Johnson CP, Sarna SK, Zhu YR, Buchmann E, Bonham L, Telford GL, Roza AM, Adams MB. Delayed gastroduodenal emptying is an important mechanism for control of intestinal transit in short gut syndrome. *Am J Surg* 1996; 171:90-5.
[55] Nightingale JM, Kamm MA, van der Sijp JR, Ghatei MA, Bloom SR, Lennard-Jones JE. Gastrointestinal hormones in short bowel syndrome. Peptide YY may be the 'colonic brake' to gastric emptying. *Gut* 1996; 39:267-72.
[56] Purdum PP, Kirby DF. Short bowel syndrome: a review of the role of nutrition support. *JPEN J Parenter Enteral Nutr* 1991; 15:93-101.
[57] Stringer MD, Puntis JWL. Short bowel syndrome. *Arch Dis Child* 1995; 73:170-3.
[58] Dudrick SJ, Latifi R. Management of short-bowel syndrome. In: Kirby DF, Dudrick SJ, eds. *Practical handbook of nutrition in clinical practice*. Boca Raton: CRC Press, 1994.
[59] O'Brien DP, Nelson LA, Huang FS, Warner BW. Intestinal adaptation: structure, function, and regulation. *Semin Pediatr Surg* 2001;10:56-64.
[60] Mainoya JR. Influence of ovine growth hormone on water and NaCl absorption by the rat proximal jejunum and distal ileum. *Comp Biochem Physiol Comp Physiol.* 1982;71:477-9.
[61] Pilling GP, Cresson SL. Massive resection of small intestine in the neonatal period. Report of two successful cases and review of the literature. *Pediatrics* 1957; 19: 940-8.
[62] Kurz R, Sauer H. Treatment and metabolic findings in extreme short-bowel syndrome with 11 cm jejunal remnant. *J Pediatr Surg* 1983;18:257-63.
[63] Iacono G, Carroccio A, Montalto G, Cavataio F, Lo Cascio M, Notarbatolo A. Extreme short bowel syndrome: a case for reviewing the guidelines for predicting survival. *J Pediatr Gastroenterol Nutr* 1993;16:216-9.

[64] Coran AG, Spivak D, Teitelbaum DH. An analysis of the morbidity and mortality of short-bowel syndrome in the pediatric age group. *Eur J Pediatr Surg* 1999;9:228-30.

[65] Levine GM, Deren JJ, Yezdimir E. Small bowel resection: oral intake is the stimulus for hyperplasia. *Am. J. Dig. Dis.* 1976;21:542-6.

[66] Lentze MJ. Intestinal adaptation in short-bowel syndrome. *Eur J Pediatr* 1989;148:294-9.

[67] WilliamsonRC. Intestinal adaptation (first of two parts).Structural, functional and cytokinetic changes. *N Engl J Med* 1978;298:1393-402.

[68] Hanson WR, Osborne JW, Sharp JG. Compensation by the residual intestine after intestinal resection in the rat. I. Influence of amount of tissue removed. *Gastroenterology* 1977;72: 692-700.

[69] Hanson WR, Osborne JW, Sharp JG. Compensation by the residual intestine after intestinal resection in the rat. II. Influence of postoperative time interval. *Gastroenterology* 1977;72: 701-5.

[70] Kerr JF, Wyllie AH, Currie AR. Apoptosis: a basic biological phenomenon with wide-ranging implications in tissue kinetics. *Br J Cancer* 1972;26:239-57.

[71] Fan XQ, Guo YJ: Apoptosis in oncology. *Cell Res* 2001;11:1-7.

[72] Nicholson DW, Ali A, Thornberry NA, Vaillancourt JP, Ding CK, Gallant M, Gareau Y, Griffin PR, Labelle M, Lazebnik YA, et al. Identification and inhibition of the ICE/CED-3 protease necessary for mammalian apoptosis. *Nature* 1995; 376:37-43.

[73] Boise LH, Gottschalk AR, Quintans J, Thompson CB. Bcl-2 and Bcl-2-related proteins in apoptosis regulation. *Curr Top Microbiol Immunol* 1995; 200:107-121

[74] Que FG, Gores GJ. Cell death by apoptosis: basic concepts and disease relevance for the gastroenterologist. *Gastroenterology* 1996;110:1238-43.

[75] Jarboe MD, Juno RJ, Bernal NP, Knott AW, Zhang Y, Erwin CR, Warner BW: Bax deficiency rescues resection-induced enterocyte apoptosis in mice with perturbed EGF receptor function. *Surgery* 2004;136:121-6.

[76] Williamson RC . Intestinal adaptation (second of two parts) . Mechanisms of control. *N Engl J Med* 1978;298:1444-50.

[77] Hanson WR, Osborne JW, Sharp JG. Compensation by the residual intestine after intestinal resection in the rat -influence of amount of tissue removed. *Gastroenterology* 1977;72:692-700.

[78] Tavakkolizadeh A,WhangEE. Understanding and augmenting human intestinal adaptation: a call for more clinical research. *JPEN J Parenter Enteral Nutr* 2002;26:251-5.
[79] HinesOJ,BilchikAJ,ZinnerMJ. Adaptation of the Na+/glucose co-transporter following intestinal resection. *J Surg Res* 1994;57:22-7.
[80] Menge H, Grafe M, Lorenz-Meyer H , Riecken EO. The influence of food intake on the development of structural and functional adaptation following ileal resection in the rat. *Gut* 1975;16:468-72.
[81] Rubin DC, Swietlicki EA,Wang JL. Enterocytic gene expression in intestinal adaptation: evidence for a specific cellular response. *Am J Physiol* 1996;270:G143-52.
[82] Sukhotnik I, Gork AS, Chen M. Effect of low fat diet on lipid absorption and fatty-acid transport following bowel resection. *Pediatr Surg Int* 2001;17:25964.
[83] Thiesen A, Wild GE, Tappenden KA. Intestinal resection and steroid-associated alterations in gene expression were not accompanied by changes in lipid uptake. *Digestion* 2002;66:112-20.
[84] Hart MH, Grandjean CJ, Park JH. Essential fatty acid deficiency and postresection mucosalad aptation in the rat. *Gastroenterology* 1988;94:682-7.
[85] Booth IW, Lander AD. Short bowel syndrome. *Bailliere's Clin Gastroenterol* 1998;12:739-72.
[86] Park JHY, Grandjean CJ, Hart MH, Vanderhoof JA. Effects of dietary linoleic acid on mucosal adaptation after small bowel resection. *Digestion* 1989;44:57-65.
[87] Sukhotnik I, Mor-Vaknin N, Drongowski RA, Miselevich I, Coran AG, Harmon CM. Effect of dietary fat on early morphological intestinal adaptation in a rat with short Bowel syndrome. *Pediatr Surg Int* 2004;20:419-24.
[88] Sukhotnik I, Gork AS, Chen M, Drongowski RA, Coran AG, Harmon CM. Effect of low fat diet on lipid absorption and fatty-acid transport following bowel resection. *Pediatr Surg Int* 2001;17:259-64.
[89] Welters CF, Dejong CH, Deutz NE. Intestinal function and metabolism in the early adaptive phase after massive small bowel resection in the rat. *J Pediatr Surg* 2001;36:1746-51.
[90] Klimberg VS, Souba WW, Salloum RM, et al. Intestinal glutamine metabolism after massive small bowel resection. *Am J Surg* 1990;159:27-32.

[91] Deutz NE, Dejong CH, Athanasas G. Partial enterectomy in the rat does not diminish muscle glutamine production. *Metabolism* 1992;41:1343-50.

[92] Alavi K,KatoY,YuD. Enteral glutamine does not enhance the effects of hepatocyte growth factor in short bowel syndrome. *J Pediatr Surg* 1998;33:1666-9.

[93] Sukhotnik I, Lerner A, Sabo E, Krausz MM, Siplovich L, Coran AG, Mogilner J, Shiloni E. Effects of enteral arginine supplementation on the structural intestinal adaptation in a rat model of short bowel syndrome. *Dig Dis Sci* 2003;48:1346-51.

[94] Czernichow B, Nsi-Emvo E, Galluser M. Enteral supplementation with ornithine alpha-ketoglutarate improves the early adaptive response to resection. *Gut* 1997;40:67-72.

[95] Swartz-Basile DA, Wang L, Tang Y, Pitt HA, Rubin DC, Levin MS. Vitamin A deficiency inhibits intestinal adaptation by modulating apoptosis, proliferation, and enterocyte migration. *Am J Physiol Gastrointest Liver Physiol* 2003;285:G424-32.

[96] Nightingale JM, Kamm MA, van der Sijp JR, Ghatei MA, Bloom SR, Lennard-Jones JE. Gastrointestinal hormones in short bowel syndrome. Peptide YY may be the 'colonic brake' to gastric emptying. *Gut* 1996;39:267-72.

[97] Drucker DJ. Gut adaptation and the glucagon-like peptides. *Gut* 2002;50:428-35.

[98] Litvak DA, Hellmich MR, Evers BM, Banker NA, Townsend CM Jr. Glucagon-like peptide 2 is a potent growth factor for small intestine and colon. *J Gastrointest Surg* 1998;2:146-50.

[99] Martin GR, Wallace LE, Hartmann B, Holst JJ, Demchyshyn L, Toney K, Sigalet DL. Nutrient stimulated GLP-2 release and crypt cell proliferation in experimental short bowel syndrome. Am. J. Physiol. Gastrointest. *Liver Physiol* 2005;288:G431-8.

[100] Jeppesen PB, Hartmann B, Thulesen J. Elevated plasma glucagon-like peptide 1 and 2 concentrations in ileum resected short bowel patients with a preserved colon. *Gut* 2000;47:370-6.

[101] Jeppesen PB, Hartmann B, Thulesen J. Glucagon-likepeptide2 improves nutrient absorption and nutritional status in short-bowel patients with no colon. *Gastroenterology* 2001;120:806–15.

[102] Uluutku AH, Akin ML, Kurt Y, Yucel E, Cermik H, Avsar K, Celenk T. Bombesin in short bowel syndrome. *J Invest Surg* 2004; 17:135-41.

[103] Sukhotnik I, Slijper N, Karry R, Shaoul R, Coran AG, Lurie M, Shiloni E, Mogilner JG. Bombesin stimulates enterocyte turnover following massive small bowel resection in a rat. *Pediatr Surg Int* 2007;23:397-404.

[104] Bell-Anderson KS, Bryson JM. Leptin as a potential treatment for obesity: progress to date. *Treat Endocrinol* 2004; 3:11-18.

[105] Paracchini V, Pedotti P, Taioli E.Genetics of leptin and obesity: a HuGE review. *Am J Epidemiol* 2005;162:101-14.

[106] Chaudhary M, Mandir N, FitzGerald AJ, Howard JK, Lord GM, Ghatei MA, Bloom SR, Goodlad RA. Starvation, leptin and epithelial cell proliferation in the gastrointestinal tract of the mouse. *Digestion* 2000; 61:223-9.

[107] Sukhotnik I, Vadasz Z, Coran AG, Lurie M, Shiloni E, Hatoum OA, Mogilner JG. Effect of leptin on intestinal re-growth following massive small bowel resection in rat. *Pediatr Surg Int* 2006;22:9-15.

[108] Sukhotnik I, Khateeb K, Krausz MM, Sabo E, Siplovich L, Coran AG, Shiloni E. Sandostatin impairs postresection intestinal adaptation in a rat model of short bowel syndrome. *Dig Dis Sci* 2002;47:2095-102.

[109] Sukhotnik I, Shiloni E, Mogilner J, Lurie M, Hirsh M, Coran AG, Krausz MM. Effect of sex and sex hormones on structural intestinal adaptation after massive small bowel resection in rats. *J Pediatr Surg* 2005;40:489-95.

[110] Shulman DI, Hu CS, Duckett G, Lavallee-Grey M. Effects of short-term growth hormone therapy in rats undergoing 75% small intestinal resection. *J Pediatr Gastroenterol Nutr* 1992;14:3-11.

[111] Mainoya JR. Influence of bovine growth hormone on water and NaCl absorption by the rat proximal jejunum and distal ileum. *Comp Biochem Physiol* 1982;71:477-9.

[112] Waitzberg DL, Cukier C, Mucerino DR. Small bowel adaptation with growth hormone and glutamine after massive resection of rat's small bowel. *Nutr Hosp* 1999;14:81-90.

[113] Fadrique B, Lopez JM, Bermudez R. Growth hormone plus high protein diet promotes adaptation after massive small bowel resection in aged rats. *Exp Gerontol* 2001;36:1727-37.

[114] Falcone RA, Stern LE, Kemp CJ, Erwin CR, Warner BW. Intestinal adaptation occurs independ of transforming growth factor-alpha. *J Ped Surg* 2000; 35: 365-70.

[115] Sukhotnik I, Yakirevich E, Coran AG , L.Siplovich, Hirsh M , Sabo E, Krausz M, Shiloni E. Effect of transforming growth factor-alpha on

intestinal adaptation in a rat model of short bowel syndrome. *J Surg Res* 2002;108:235-42.

[116] Sukhotnik I, Mogilner JG, Shaoul R, Karry R, Lieber M, Suss-Toby E, Ure BN, Coran AG. Responsiveness of intestinal epithelial cell turnover to TGF-α after bowel resection in a rat is correlated with EGF receptor expression along the villus-crypt axis. *Ped Surg International* 2008; 24: 21-8.

[117] Lund PK. Molecular basis of intestinal adaptation: the role of the insulin-like growth factor system. *Ann N Y Acad Sci* 1998;859:18-36.

[118] Wiren M, Adrian TE, Arnelo U, Permert J, Staab P, Larsson J. An increase in mucosal insulin-like growth factor II content in postresection rat intestine suggests autocrine or paracrine growth stimulation. *Scand. J. Gastroenterol* 1998; 33: 1080-6.

[119] Ziegler TR, Mantell MP, Chow JC, Rombeau JL, Smith RJ. Gut adaptation and the insulin-like growth factor system: regulation by glutamine and IGF-1 administration. *Am J Physiol* 1996; 271 : G866-G75.

[120] Sukhotnik I, Shehadeh N, Shamir R , Bejar J, Bernshteyn A, Mogilner JG. Oral insulin enhances intestinal re-growth following massive small bowel resection in rat. *Dig Dis Sci* 2005;50:2379-85.

[121] Ben Lulu S, Coran AG, Mogilner JG, Shamir R, Shehadeh N, Sukhotnik I. Oral insulin stimulates intestinal epithelial cell turnover in correlation with insulin-receptor expression along the villus-crypt axis in a rat model of short bowel syndrome. *Pediatr Surg Int* 2010;26:37-44.

[122] Shamir R, Kolacek S, Koletzko S, Tavori I, Bader D, Litmanovitz I, Flidel-Rimon O, Marks KA, Sukhotnik I, Shehadeh N. Oral insulin supplementation in pediatric short bowel disease. A pilot observational study. *J Pediatr Gastroenterol Nutr JPGN* 2009; 49:108-111.

[123] Wildhaber BE, Yang H, Teitelbaum DH. Keratinocyte growth factor decreases total parenteral nutrition-induced apoptosis in mouse intestinal epithelium via Bcl-2. *J. Pediatr. Surg* 2003 ;38:92-6.

[124] Roberts AB, Sporn MB. Physiological actions and clinical applications of transforming growth factor-beta (TGF-beta). *Growth Factors* 1993; 8:1-9.

[125] Massaguè J. TGFβ signaling: receptors, transducers, and mad proteins. *Cell* 1996; 85:947-50.

[126] Sukhotnik I, Mogilner JG, Ben Lulu S, Bashenko Y, Shaoul R, Chemodanov E, Coran AG. Nutritional supplementation with transforming growth factor-beta (TGF-β) inhibits intestinal adaptation

after massive small bowel resection in a rat. *Ped Surg International* 2011;27:211-6.

[127] Sukhotnik I, Mogilner J, Pollak Y , Blumenfeld S, Bejar J, Coran AG. Platelet-derived growth factor-alpha (PDGF-α) stimulates intestinal epithelial cell turnover after massive small bowel resection in a rat. *American Journal of Physiology: GI & Liver* 2012;302:G1274-81.

In: Short Bowel Syndrome in Children
Editor: Igor Sukhotnik
ISBN: 978-1-62948-518-8

Chapter IV

Mortality and Morbidity of Short Bowel Syndrome

A. G. Coran, M.D. and I. Sukhotnik, M.D.
University of Michigan, Section of Pediatric Surgery,
Mott Children's Hospital, Ann Arbor,
MI and Technion-Israel Institute of Technology,
The Ruth and Bruce Rappaport Faculty of Medicine,
Dept of Pediatric Surgery and Pathology,
Bnai Zion Medical Center, Haifa, Israel

Abstract

Short bowel syndrome (SBS) continues to be an important clinical problem due to its high mortality and morbidity as well as to its devastating socioeconomic effects. The medical management and nutritional support of a patient with SBS is complex and requires a multidisciplinary approach with the surgeon, gastroenteroliogist, pharmacist and dietitian working together. The common causes of death in this population have been related to sepsis or intestinal failure associated liver disease. The use of parenteral and enteral nutrition in our daily practice has dramatically improved the outcomes during the past three decades. More than 90% of infants and children now survive after extensive small bowel resection in the neonatal period. Effectively caring for SBS patients and their families is a complex task that is best carried out in a coordinated, multi-disciplinary setting. The benefits of a multi-disciplinary approach include the stream-lined diagnosis and treatment, strengthened communication with families and the care teams, amalgamation of expert care, a holistic approach to patients, consistent follow up and continuity of patient care.

Keywords: Short bowel syndrome, intestinal failure, intestinal failure associated liver disease, risk factors; morbidity, mortality, rehabilitation, survival, prognosis, intestinal rehabilitation program

As a result of marked improvements in both critical care and nutritional support, the pediatric surgeon is now caring for an increasing number of neonates and infants with the short-bowel syndrome (SBS). Pediatric intestinal failure is a complex clinical problem which is associated with high patient mortality and morbidity. The etiology of this syndrome is multifactorial and includes a host of congenital as well as acquired etiologies. Although definitions of the SBS have ranged from less than 70% of normal small-bowel length to a very short length of small bowel (<10% of normal length), the absolute length of bowel appears to be a less critical factor than the absolute absorptive capacity of the remaining small bowel, the presence or absence of an ileocecal valve, as well as the specific small bowel remaining (ileum or jejunum) [1,2]. The functional consequences of short bowel syndrome depend on the length, surface area, and the site of the resected small intestine. Preservation of ileum appears to be more important than preservation of jejunum because the ileum can often adapt and perform much of the jejunal absorptive functions. Additionally, the majority of small bowel growth occurs in the third trimester of pregnancy; therefore, premature infants appear to have a greater capacity to gain additional small-bowel growth after resection than full-term newborns or older children [3]. The nutritional support of a child with the short-bowel syndrome is complex and requires a multidisciplinary approach with the pediatric surgeon, pediatric gastroenterologist, pharmacist and dietitian working together. The benefits of a multi-disciplinary approach include the amalgamation of expert care, a holistic approach to patients, stream-lined diagnosis and treatment, strengthened communication with both families and the care teams, consistent follow up and continuity of patient care. The care of such an infant can be divided into three stages [4]. The first stage of care begins after resuscitation of the patient in the post-operative period or at the time the diagnosis of short bowel syndrome has been made. The syndrome is associated with increased gastric output, due to a loss of intrinsic intestinal negative feedback and increased stool output, which often leads to fluid and electrolyte shifts and losses of nutrients and trace elements. During this time a permanent silastic central venous catheter (e.g. *Broviac)* needs to be inserted. Since the child will need long-term venous access, each access site must be carefully cared for and protected. The child's main or sole caloric source will be via the parenteral route for a considerable period of time. Nevertheless, enteral feedings should be initiated within 1 to 2 weeks after the onset of the short-bowel syndrome. Enteral feedings will both stimulate small-bowel adaptation and prevent the development of parenteral nutrition-associated cholestasis. The ideal enteral solution should be isotonic, or nearly isotonic as this will be better tolerated by the gastrointestinal tract. The protein source should be predominately di- and tripeptides, since this source of protein is most easily and efficiently absorbed [5,6]. The solution should have a fair amount of medium chain triglycerides, as this source of fat is well absorbed through the basolateral wall of the intestinal enterocytes. However, medium chain triglycerides contain no essential fatty acids; therefore, these fats cannot be the sole source of lipids in these patients. In infants, we prefer to initiate feedings with Pregestamil (Mead Johnson), and in children over one year of age we generally utilize Petamen Junior. High stool output is associated with excessive losses of zinc; thus, zinc supplementation, above that normally required, should be provided in the parenteral nutrition solution. Finally, the loss of sodium and bicarbonate in such patients can be dramatic and total body sodium depletion has been shown to be associated with failure to thrive, despite the administration of adequate amounts of calories [7,8]. A simple way to detect such a deficit is to measure spot urine sodium. Urine sodium of less than 10 meq/l may well indicate total body sodium depletion and supplementation via the oral route should be given on a daily basis. During the second phase of support, a more stabilized state has been reached, at which point careful monitoring of the patient's nutritional status is very important. Electrolytes, liver function tests and assessment of protein status (total protein, albumin and total iron-binding capacity) should be done initially and on a weekly basis. Fat-soluble vitamin levels should be assessed approximately every six months to assure that adequate amounts are being absorbed. Serum levels of vitamins A, D and E can be assayed. A prothrombin time will be indicative of vitamin K levels. Patients with a significant loss of the terminal ileum should have a vitamin B12 level assessed on a yearly basis. Supplementation of fat-soluble vitamins, if depleted, should also be carried out. The child's stool should intermittently be assessed for pH, reducing substances and qualitative fecal fats. A stool pH~5.5 or a reducing substance level greater than one half percent indicates malabsorption of carbohydrates. Elevation in fecal fats will suggest fat malabsorption, which may require modification of the child's enteral diet (i. e. increase the percent of medium-chain triglycerides). Formulas with sucrose as the carbohydrate will not yield a positive reducing substance test despite carbohydrate malabsorption. The final phase of nutritional support consists of weaning the patient from parenteral nutrition. During this stage, which may last from months to years, a variety of factors must also be monitored. These include an assurance that the child will develop normal suck and swallow reflexes and not develop an aversion to oral feedings. Also, the child should be monitored for normal length and weight gain. Finally, patients with an intact colon should be evaluated for the development of renal oxalate stones, and, thus, should avoid a high oxalate diet.

Until 30 years ago, the prognosis after extensive bowel resection was poor, especially in the neonatal period. The survival of pediatric patients with intestinal failure has traditionally been dismal, with greater than 40% mortality. The common causes of death in this population have been related to sepsis or end stage liver disease from intestinal failure associated liver disease (IFALD). The onset of parenteral and enteral feeding in daily practice has transformed the outcome during the past decades [9-16] (Table 1). More than 90% of infants and children now survive after extensive small bowel resection in the neonatal period [17]. A study from the Province of Ontario, Canada, estimated the overall mortality rate in 40 neonatal SBS patients to be 37.5% with hepatic failure being responsible for 60% of SBS deaths [18]. A recent survey of 87 children who had undergone extensive small bowel resection as neonates, followed up over a 15-year period [9] showed an overall survival of 89.7%. Risk factors thought to contribute to the high morbidity and mortality of SBS include the length of remaining small bowel, sepsis, loss of the ileo-cecal valve (ICV), and development of PN associated cholestasis [19-21]. The duration of PN dependency varies according to the intestinal length and the presence of the ICV. The conjugated bilirubin (more than 2.5 mg/dL) is the strongest predictor of survival [22].

In another study, the presence of an ICV did not correlate with successful PN weaning but did affect the mean duration of PN therapy. Patients with 40 cm or less of initial small bowel spend a longer time on PN and have a lower weaning rate than those with longer bowel. The ratio of initial small bowel length to birth weight does not correlate with the duration of PN therapy in survivors successfully weaned from PN [10].

The institution of an aggressive protocol of advancing enteric feeds, oral antibiotic prophylaxis for bacterial overgrowth, fish oil-based lipid use, and the STEP procedure for dilated bowel has resulted in an increase in survival and a remarkable improvement in liver function in the pediatric SBS population [23]. SBS with a very short remaining gut (less than 40 cm) has a high mortality, but 1/3 of these patients will adapt after as long as 5 years [24].

Table 1. Prognosis of short bowel syndrome

Series	Year	No of patients	Range of remaining small bowel length (cm)	Survival	Percent of surviving patients adapted (No TPN)
Goulet	1991	16	22-98	82	86
Weber	1991	87	48	94	67
Georgeson	1992	52	8-100	83	75
Guarino	2003	109	NR	94	42
Sigalet	2006	20	87±47	100	82
Pakarinen	2009	20	33±21	90	60
Martinez	2011	63	<40cm	67	27
Khalil	2012	27	36	93	78

Recently, an interest in "rehabilitating" the intestinal remnant in these patients has surfaced. Use of enteral glutamine, high-fiber diet and systemic growth hormone has been tried in patients on long-term TPN. A three-week course of this therapy apparently resulted in improved caloric absorption from the intestine and decreased stool output [25]. Experience in children, however, is lacking and further work in this age group will be needed to confirm these findings. Additionally, attempts at lengthening the intestine in children with short-bowel syndrome have met with reasonable results in some children, both by prolonging transit time and improving the ineffective peristalsis associated with the dilated intestine [26,27]. Despite the above-described aggressive medical and surgical management, morbidity and mortality are not uncommon in this syndrome. An early study of our group of short-bowel syndrome (SBS) patients treated over a 10-year period identified which associated factors may contribute to patient morbidity and mortality [28]. All infants and children managed at the C. S. Mott Children's Hospital with the diagnosis of short-bowel syndrome between June, 1983 and May, 1993, were identified. All hospital and clinical charts were reviewed. Our definition of SBS was a loss of

70% or more of total small-bowel length. The following were the potential risk factors for morbidity and mortality in these children with SBS: catheter-related sepsis, TPN-associated cholestasis, growth and nutrition, small-bowel length and presence of an ileocecal valve. Intra-venous lines were utilized in all patients and were in place for a mean of 614 days. A total of 73 catheter-related infections occurred and each child suffered from a mean of 7.4/1000 catheter-days. Only 2 of the 19 patients remained infection-free. All infections were confirmed by a positive blood culture. Successful treatment of line sepsis was accomplished in 94% of gram negative and 90% of gram-positive infections. Despite apparent eradication of an organism, the same organism was found with a subsequent catheter infection in 38 septic episodes from 11 patients. Importantly, the number of septic episodes was not significantly associated with patient mortality. Nor were the number of septic episodes significantly greater in any of the subgroups of patients previously mentioned. The only risk factor associated with increased sepsis rates was bowel ·length. The number of septic episodes was statistically higher in those patients with intestinal lengths less than 30cm (10.4 vs. 5.6 episodes). Because of this, we speculated that the shorter the length of small intestine the greater the incidence of sepsis. However, when we expressed line sepsis as the number of infections per 1000 catheter days and compared them to the length of small intestine, the number of septic episodes actually appeared to increase with increasing bowel length. Direct bilirubin levels were predictive indicator of patient survival. Sixty-one percent of children developed a hyperbilirubinernia of ~2.5 mg/dl. Of these children with hyperbilirubinemia, 36% were non-survivors. In several patients, the hyperbilirubinernia was transient, but 67 % of children died if they had a direct bilirubin of >4 mg/dl of ~6 months duration. Other liver function tests, including SGOT, SGPT, LDH and Alkaline phosphatase, did not significantly correlate with adverse outcome. Bilirubin levels in the non-survivors rose quickly and a significant distinction between survivors and non-survivors became evident within the first 3 months after the development of SBS. Serum albumin levels were routinely measured. A statistical difference was noted in albumin levels between survivors and non-survivors. A similarly significant difference was seen in serum total protein between these two groups. Growth as measured by body weight was also poor in non-survivors. Four of the 5 non-survivors were at or below the 5th percentile for weight, whereas mean growth in the remaining patients was normal. Mean small intestinal length was 46cm. Although mean length of bowel was greater in those children weaned from TPN, no statistical difference was noted between the groups. Those patients who successfully weaned from

TPN had intact ileocecal valves more frequently than those who did not (60% vs 29%); however, this difference was not significant. Furthermore, patient survival was not influenced by the presence of an ileocecal valve. Six of the 7 patients with an ileocecal valve are survived, compared with 8 of 12 patients without an ileocecal valve.

A recent systematic review was performed on Medline, Pubmed, and Embase conference proceedings and trial registries [29]. All study designs comparing intestinal rehabilitation programs (IRP) to traditional management of pediatric intestinal failure were included in a meta-analysis. Fifteen independent studies were included. Compared to historical controls, implementation of an IRP resulted in a reduction in septic episodes (0.3 vs. 0.5 event/month) and an increase in overall patient survival (22% vs. 42%). Non-significant improvements were seen in weaning from PN, incidence of IFALD, and relative risk of liver transplantation. Other outcomes reported included a reduction in calories from parenteral nutrition (100% vs. 32%–56%), earlier surgical/transplant evaluation, and improved coordination of patient care.

In summary, although patient survival in infants and children with SBS has improved significantly in recent years, the morbidity of SBS remains strikingly high, and many patients who do not wean off TPN eventually die. Factors associated with decreased survival are a persistently elevated direct bilirubin, low albumin and low total protein levels. The majority of patients' deaths are due to either liver failure or malnutrition. The risk of catheter sepsis appears to increase with increasing lengths of small intestine. The ability to wean from TPN is associated with bowel length or the presence of an ileocecal valve. This suggests that it is the remaining functional integrity of the intestine that is of greatest importance rather than outward appearance of the intestine. Improvement in and prevention of these risk factors may improve overall patient survival in the SBS. Multi-disciplinary teams are believed to be the best approach to successful and integrated care of children with SBS. Several studies listed in this chapter have reported significant subjective benefits since the introduction of intestinal rehabilitation programs.

References

[1] Kurkclwbasclle A, Rowe M, Sl1lith S. Adaptation in short bowel syndrome: Reassessing old limits. *J Pediatr Surg* 1993; 28: 1069-1071.

[2] Wilmore D. Faetors eOlTelating with a sueeessful outeome following extensive intestinal resection in newbom infants. *J Pecliatr* 1972; 80: 88-95.

[3] Parekh NR, Steiger E. Short bowel syndrome. *Curr Treat Options Gastroenterol 2007*;10:10-23.

[4] Dudrick SJ, Latifi R. Management of short-bowel syndrome. In: Kirby DF, Dudrick SJ, eds. *Practical handbook of nutrition in clinical practice.* Boca Raton: CRC Press, 1994.

[5] Woolf GM, Miller C, Kurian R, Jeejeebhoy KN. Diet for patients with a short bowel: high fat or high carbohydrate? *Gastroenterology* 1983; 84:823-8.

[6] Woolf GM, Miller C, Kurian R, Jeejeebhoy KN. Nutritional absorption in short bowel syndrome: evaluation of fluid, calories, and divalent cation requirements. *Dig Dis Sci* 1987; 32:8-15.

[7] Bower TR. Pril1gle KC, Soper RT: Soclium defieit eausing deereased weight gain and metabolie aeidosis in infants with ileostomy. *J Pediatr Surg* 1988; 23: 567-572.

[8] Sacher P, Hirsig F, Gresser F, Spitz L. The importance of oral sodium replaeement in ileostomy patients. *Prog Pecliatr Surg* 1989; 24:116-131.

[9] Goulet O, Baglin-Gobet S, Jais JP, Michel JL, Jan D, Ricour C. Outcome and long-term growth after extensive small bowel resection in the neonatal period: a survey of 87 children. *Eur J Pediatr Surg* 2005;15:95–101.

[10] Georgeson KE, Breaux CW. Outcome and intestinal adaptation in neonatal short bowel syndrome. *J Pediatr Surg* 1992; 27:344-350.

[11] Cowles RA, Ventura KA, Martinez M, et al. Reversal of intestinal failure-associated liver disease in infants and children on parenteral nutrition: experience with 93 patients at a referral center for intestinal rehabilitation. *J Pediatr Surg* 2010;45:84-88.

[12] Javid PJ, Malone FR, Reyes J. The experience of a regional pediatric intestinal failure program: successful outcomes from intestinal rehabilitation. *Am J Surg* 2010;199:676-679.

[13] Guarino A, De Marco G. and the Italian National Network for Pediatric Intestinal Failure. Natural history of intestinal failure, investigated through a national network-based approach. *J Pediatr Gastroenterol Nutr* 2003;37:136-141.

[14] Hess RA, Welch KB, Brown PI. Survival outcomes of pediatric intestinal failure patients: analysis of factors contributing to improved survival over the past two decades. *J Surg Res* 2011;170:27-31.

[15] Colomb V, Dabbas-Tyan M, Taupin P. Long term outcome of children receiving home parenteral nutrition: a 20-year single-center experience in 302 patients. *J Pediatr Gastroenterol Nutr* 2007;44:347-353.
[16] Khalil BA, Ba'ath ME, Aziz A. Intestinal rehabilitation and bowel reconstructive surgery: improved outcomes in children with short bowel syndrome. *J Pediatr Gastroenterol Nutr* 2012;54:505-509.
[17] Pakarinen MP, Koivusalo AI, Rintala RJ. Outcomes of intestinal failure-a comparison between children with short bowel and dysmotile intestine. *J Pediatr Surg* 2009;44:2139-2144.
[18] Wales PW, de Silva N, Kim J. Neonatal short bowel syndrome: population-based estimates of incidence and mortality rates. *J Pediatr Surg* 2004; 39:690–695.
[19] Bueno J, Guiterrez J, Mazariegos GV, Abu-Elmagd K, Madariaga J, Ohwada S, Kocoshis S, Reyes J. Analysis of patients with longitudinal intestinal lengthening procedure referred for intestinal transplantation. *J Pediatr Surg* 2001;36:178 –183.
[20] Ziegler MM. Short bowel syndrome: remedial features that influence outcome and the duration of parenteral nutrition. *J Pediatr* 1997;131: 335–336.
[21] Teitelbaum DH. Parenteral nutrition-associated cholestasis. *Curr Opin Pediatr* 1997;9:270–275.
[22] Spencer AU, Neaga A, West B, Safran J, Brown P, Btaiche I, Kuzma-O'Reilly B, Teitelbaum DH. Pediatric short bowel syndrome: redefining predictors of success. *Ann Surg* 2005;242:403-409.
[23] Sigalet D, Boctor D, Robertson M, Lam V, Brindle M, Sarkhosh K, Driedger L, Sajedi M. Improved outcomes in paediatric intestinal failure with aggressive prevention of liver disease. *Eur J Pediatr Surg* 2009;19:348-353.
[24] Martínez M, Fabeiro M, Dalieri M, Barcellandi P, Prozzi M, Hernández J, Alberti M, Fernández A. Outcome and survival of pediatric Short Bowel Syndrome (SBS). *Nutr Hosp* 2011;26:239-242.
[25] Byme TA, Morrissey TB, Nattakom TV, Ziegler TR, Will1lOre DW. Growth hormone, glutamine, and a moclified cliet enhanee nutrient absorption in patients with severe short bowel syndrome. *J Parenteral and Enteral Nutrition* 1995; 19: 296-302.
[26] Bianchi A. Intestinal loop lengthening - a teehnique for inereasing small intestinallength. *J Pecliatr Surg* 1980; 15: 145-151.
[27] Pokorny W, Fowler C. Isoperistaltie intestinallengthening for short bowel syndrome. *Surg Gyn Obst* 1991;172: 39-43.

[28] Coran AG, Spivak D, Teitelbaum DH. An analysis of the morbidity and mortality of short-bowel syndrome in the pediatric age group. *Eur J Pediatr Surg* 1999;9:228-230.

[29] Stanger JD, Oliveira C, Blackmore C, Avitzur Y, Wales PW. The impact of multi-disciplinary intestinal rehabilitation programs on the outcome of pediatric patients with intestinal failure: a systematic review and meta-analysis. *J Pediatr Surg* 2013;48:983-992.

In: Short Bowel Syndrome in Children
Editor: Igor Sukhotnik
ISBN: 978-1-62948-518-8

Chapter V

Intestinal Failure-Associated Liver Disease

Ron Shaoul*, M.D.

Pediatric Gastroenterology Unit, Rambam Medical Center, Technion, Faculty of Medicine, Haifa, Israel

Abstract

Total parenteral nutrition (TPN)-associated cholestasis (PNAC) and intestinal failure-associated liver disease (IFALD) is a significant life-threatening complication in children with short bowel syndrome (SBS). It has been estimated that IFALD develops in 40% to 60% of infants who require long-term TPN for intestinal failure and 15% to 40% of adults on home parenteral nutrition. The cause of IFALD is thought to be multifactorial. Predisposing factors include early premature birth, very low birth weight, birth weight small for gestational age, early septic infection, impaired bile acid recirculation, delayed/limited enteral feeding, long duration of parenteral nutrition, phytosterols, lipid peroxides etc. In the current chapter the incidence of PNAC/IFALD in children receiving TPN and the efficacy of measures to prevent/treat PNAC/IFALD have been reviewed.

* Correspondence/reprints requests: Ron Shaoul, MD, Director, Pediatric Gastroenterology and Nutrition Unit, Meyer Children's Hospital of Haifa, Rambam Medical Center, POB 9602, Haifa 31096, Israel. Email: shaoul_r@012.net.il.

Background

Intestinal failure (IF) is a condition of malabsorption that is due to reduction of functional intestinal mass necessary for adequate digestion and absorption for nutrient, fluid and growth requirements [1,2]. It is often the result of dysmotility, surgical resection, a congenital defect or disease-associated loss of absorption. Children with intestinal failure (IF) suffer from insufficient intestinal length or function, making them dependent on parenteral nutrition (PN) for growth and survival and they endure significant mortality and morbidity [3]. Although the introduction of PN has altered the outcome for neonates and infants with IF, liver dysfunction is commonly encountered, especially in neonates [4,5]. Although abnormal liver function tests associated with short-term parenteral nutrition are usually benign and transient, liver dysfunction in both children and adults receiving long-term parenteral nutrition can progress to end-stage liver disease and liver failure. Management of IF primarily focuses on intestinal rehabilitation using a multidisciplinary approach including nutritional, pharmacologic and surgical interventions to achieve the goal of full enteral nutrition (EN) [2,6].

There is an increasing awareness over the recent decades for intestinal failure associated liver disease (IFALD) in both children and adults. It has been estimated that IFALD develops in 40% to 60% of infants who require long-term total parenteral nutrition (TPN) for intestinal failure and 15% to 40% of adults on home parenteral nutrition [4]. The most effective treatment for IFALD is increasing enteral caloric intake while reducing PN, but this process is often impossible when intestinal function is poor [2]. Data from the Pediatric Intestinal Failure Consortium suggests that enteral autonomy may require years to achieve [7,8].

Diagnosis

Clinical Features

Children in whom the diagnosis of IFALD is considered should be carefully examined for signs of liver disease. The clinical features include jaundice, hepatomegaly, splenomegaly, ascites, edema, spider nevi, palmar erythema, and dilated veins in the anterior abdominal wall (caput medusae) [9].

Laboratory Studies

The diagnosis of IFALD has historically been established by routine biochemical tests of hepatic function [9]. These tests include conjugated/direct bilirubin (cholestasis), albumin and international normalized ratio (INR; hepatic synthetic function), gamma-glutamyl transferase (GGT; cholestasis), alanine aminotransferase (ALT; hepatic injury), platelet count, and absolute neutrophil count (ANC; portal hypertension). These laboratory values are essential in the diagnosis of IFALD, commonly defined as a direct bilirubin of greater than or equal to 2.0 mg/dL. An increase in the conjugated bilirubin is often the earliest sign of IFALD and is a surrogate for cholestasis as well as a relative indicator of liver excretory function [9].

Kaufman et al. [10] examined the hypothesis that early trends in common blood tests may delineate risks of liver failure in infants with parenteral nutrition-associated liver disease from short bowel syndrome. They found that progressively worsening hyperbilirubinemia, thrombocytopenia, and hypoalbuminemia were all independent predictors of liver failure; for every 1 mg/dL increase in the serum bilirubin, the odds of developing liver failure increased by 20%; for every 1000/mL decrease in platelet count, the odds of developing liver failure increased by 1%; and for every 1.0 g/dL decrease in albumin, the odds of liver failure increased by 75%. Recently, Diaz et al. [11] have showed that aspartate aminotransferase (AST) to platelet ratio index (APRI) values significantly predicts cirrhosis but not fibrosis in pediatric patients with IFALD.

Clinical Spectrum and Prognosis

The clinical spectrum of IFALD includes hepatic steatosis, cholestasis, fibrosis, and, ultimately, progression to hepatic cirrhosis with portal hypertension and end-stage liver disease [4,5]. Studies have shown that liver disease in patients on long-term PN is strongly correlated with survival. In a cohort of 78 children with SBS, the survival rate among those with cholestasis (conjugated bilirubin >2mg/dL), was close to 20% compared with 80% in those without cholestasis [12]. In addition, the degree of liver dysfunction has also been correlated with outcome. A recent study evaluating a cohort of 66 patients with IFALD reported that, although 38% of infants with a maximum conjugated bilirubin greater than or equal to 10 mg/dL died or were referred for intestinal transplantation, only 7% of infants with a maximum conjugated bilirubin less than 10 mg/dL died during the first year of life [13]. Other studies report that the mortality of patients with end-stage liver disease while on PN approaches 100%, as does the mortality of neonates with IFALD within a year of diagnosis if they are unable to be weaned off PN or fail to receive a liver/small bowel transplant [14]. Overall, approximately 15% of patients with IFALD progress to end stage liver disease requiring either isolated or combined liver–small bowel transplantation [9,12,14-16].

Pathogenesis of IFALD

The cause of IFALD is thought to be multifactorial. A major predisposing factor is hepatic immaturity, as shown by the different prevalence and presentation of parenteral nutrition-associated liver disease in pediatric and in adult patients and by the increased prevalence in infants with early premature birth, very low birth weight, or birth weight small for gestational age [17-19] and long duration of TPN [4]. Experimental studies have shown that short-term fasting has several metabolic and endocrine consequences on intestinal and liver function. Levels of gastrointestinal hormones, such as gastrin, motilin, glucose-dependent insulinotropic polypeptide, secretin, pancreatic polypeptide, glucagons, and vasoactive intestinal peptide, are reduced in patients on TPN who are not being enterally fed [4,20]. This may lead to reduced gallbladder contractility and the development of intestinal stasis [4,20-22]. The reduction in cholecystokinin release may influence gallbladder size and contractility and cause the development of biliary sludge [4,23].

Bishay et al. [24] retrospectively studied 87 infants requiring PN for at least 28 days. They found that IFALD developed in 29 infants (33%). IFALD was managed medically in all but 2 patients who underwent intestinal elongation. None were referred for intestinal or liver transplant. IFALD resolved in 17 (59%) of cases. Severity of IFALD was significantly associated with duration of PN and female sex. Recently, Pichler et al. [25] reviewed all long-term IF patients over 4 years for the possible predisposing factors of age, diagnosis, PN lipid, sepsis, length of PN treatment and length of hospitalisation. Outcome measures were IFALD incidence, severity and prognosis. Of 60/279 (%22) children aged 0-18 years who developed IFALD, 13 (5%) progressed to type 3 end stage disease. IFALD was associated with younger age ($p=0.03$), longer treatment ($p<0.001$), longer hospitalisation ($p=0.01$), surgical diagnosis ($p=0.005$) and prematurity ($p=0.03$). Interestingly, IFALD was not associated with sepsis. Intestinal surgery was associated with

IFALD independently of age (p=0.03). Survival was 86%, with three deaths attributed to IFALD (1% of all cases), all of which were surgical.

Beale et al. [26] reviewed 62 premature infants on TPN. The incidence of cholestasis was 23%, but infants receiving therapy for more than 60 days had an incidence of 80% increasing to 90% in those treated for more than 3 months. The incidence of cholestasis was 50% in infants with birth weight below1000 g but decreased to 7% if birth weight was above 1500 g. This observation has been confirmed by Beath et al. [27] who found the highest incidence in infants with less than 34-week gestation and who weighed less than 2 kg. Other reported predisposing factors associated with IFALD are: number of laparotomies, number of days on antibiotics, and delayed start to enteral feeding[4,28]. A further key risk factor for the development of IFALD is the early occurrence of severe infections, such as catheter-related septic infections, necrotizing enterocolitis, or small intestinal bacterial overgrowth (SIBO) with subsequent gram-negative sepsis [12,17-19]. Bacterial overgrowth from intestinal stasis has been related to the development of IFALD possibly because of the combination of the reduction in bile flow, the production of secondary bile salts, and sepsis from bacterial translocation [4,29]. Another documented risk factor is impaired bile acid recirculation and secretion, with increased risk in patients with loss of the distal ileum and/or the ileo-coecal valve, lack of primary bowel anastomosis, and lack of, or delayed introduction and low advancement of, enteral feeding [12,17,30]. Documented and proposed risk factors for development of IFALD are listed in table 1.

Table 1. Causes for development of IFALD

(1) Early premature birth.
(2) Very low birth weight, birth weight small for gestational age.
(3) Early septic infection (catheter infection, necrotizing enterocolitis).
(4) Impaired bile acid recirculation (short bowel syndrome with loss of the distal ileum and/or the ileocoecal valve, lack of primary bowel anastomosis).
(5) Delayed/limited enteral feeding.
(6) Long duration of parenteral nutrition.
(7) Excessive/imbalanced parenteral substrate supply.
(8) Phytosterols.
(9) Lipid peroxides.

The Role of TPN

Inadequate composition and administration of parenteral nutrition, in particular excessive and imbalanced substrate supplies, and continuous infusion with subsequent insulin/glucagon imbalance are discussed as potential further risk factors for IFALD, but considerable uncertainty remains regarding the contribution of different incriminated factors [17,30]. Recently, lipid emulsions containing fish oils as the triglyceride source were proposed to be protective in IFALD [2,17]. Until now, soybean oil, rich in omega-6 fatty acids, continues to be the main lipid source in the various intravenous lipid emulsions (ILE). Early experimental reports suggested that soybean oil-based ILE negatively influenced immunologic cell functions [31]. More recently, clinical and experimental evidence suggested a role for soybean oil-based ILE in the onset of IFALD [2]. Clinical observation showed a positive relation of the dosage of soybean oil-based lipid emulsion with the development of cholestasis in children on long-term parenteral nutrition, with occurrence of cholestatic episodes after a dosage increase, and reduction of elevated serum bilirubin levels after stopping lipid infusion or reducing the dosage [17,32] . As more evidence accumulated against soybean oil-based lipid emulsion, the development of alternative lipid emulsions, including those containing olive oil and fish oil, started to appear [2,33]. The difference among the ILEs is primarily the composition of the long-chain polyunsaturated fatty acids. An ILE that is made from fish oil contains high amounts of docosahexaenoic acid (DHA) and eicosapentaenoic acid (EPA) which have potential for an anti-inflammatory benefit. Gura et al. [34] were the first to report on the use of a fish oil based lipid emulsion as the only triglyceride source in two infants with short bowel syndrome and end stage liver disease, who showed improvement and in one case even removal from the transplant list. The same group reported their experience with 42 infants with short bowel syndrome and bilirubin above 2 mg/dl who were treated with parenteral nutrition with a lipid emulsion based on fish oil as the only triglyceride source. This group was compared with historical controls of 49 infants treated with parenteral nutrition with a higher dosage of soybean oil-based lipid emulsion. The fish oil-treated patients showed a higher rate and faster recovery from IFALD [35]. Diamond et al. [36] did a retrospective review of children with short bowel syndrome and IFALD treated in 2006 and 2007 with a combination of soybean oil emulsion and fish oil-based emulsion. Nine out of the 12 reported children patients showed complete resolution of hyperbilirubinaemia within a median of 24 weeks. A randomized controlled trial in 60 premature infants with a gestational age of no more than 34 weeks found a significantly lesser increase of plasma gGT levels in infants randomized to a lipid emulsion with a mixture of soybean, olive, coconut, and fish oils than in those receiving the control emulsion without fish oil [37]. In agreement with these observations, the results of several studies in different adult patient groups showed improved markers of liver function after the administrations of mixed lipid emulsions with some fish oil, relative to control emulsions without fish oil [17,37,38]. These observations raise the question whether emulsions with all of the triglycerides constituting fish oil are necessary to achieve a benefit in IFALD, or whether a mixture of different oil sources and added a-tocopherol might also be effective.

Lipid Dosing

Standard guidelines recommend administering lipid emulsions at a dose of less than 2.5 g/kg/d. However, a dose greater than 1 g/kg/d has been associated with the development of IFALD [2,9,32,39-41], whereas a dose less than or equal to 1 g/kg/d has been shown to be effective in preventing IFALD. Since enzymatic pathways in neonates are not adequately developed and cannot efficiently convert ALA and LA to their active moieties, DHA and AA supplementation of downstream fatty acids is extremely important [9,42,43].

Other Components

Other components of the TPN have been associated with IFALD. These include deficiency or excess of amino acids in the TPN solutions. It is possible that hepatotoxicity may be caused by a deficiency of taurine or cysteine, which are conditional essential amino acids in neonates because of the low levels of hepatic cystathionase and cysteine sulfinic decarboxylase [4,44]. Not only is taurine one of the main bile acid conjugates in the neonate, but it has been shown to increase bile flow and protect against lithocholate toxicity. Despite this, the benefits of taurine supplementation are unproven [4,45].

Elements involved in PN administration and compounding, specifically di(2-ethylhexyl) phthalate (DEHP) and aluminum, have been linked to IFALD [4,9]. DEHP is an industrial additive plasticizer present in polyvinylchloride (PVC) and infusion systems[9]. DEHP has been shown to increase oxidative stress and toxicity in preterm neonates and infants. Von Rettberg et al. [46]

found that changing to PVC free infusion systems decreased the incidence of cholestasis from 50% to 13%, and that the use of PVC infusion sets strongly correlated with the development of cholestasis. Aluminum is another element found in raw materials and incorporated into parenteral products during the manufacturing process [47]. Although aluminium toxicity is well recognized in TPN and may lead to bone disease, there is no evidence that it is implicated in TPN liver disease [4]. Chromium toxicity, secondary to TPN, has been reported in animals [4]. Both serum and urine chromium concentration levels are higher in children on long-term TPN compared with control values although there was no correlation with liver disease [4.48]. A number of studies have reported the effects of manganese toxicity in children on long-term TPN [49,50]. Children with impaired liver function had the highest manganese levels, and there was a significant correlation between whole-blood manganese levels, aspartate aminotransferase and total plasma bilirubin [49,50]. Since manganese is excreted in bile, the toxic effect may be exacerbated in cholestasis and therefore manganese levels monitoring may be important in patients with IFALD cholestasis [4].

PN Cycling

Cycling of PN involves the provision of total daily PN volume in less than 24 hours. Cycling should be adjusted as enteral intake increases and should be tailored to patient age, since neonates often have diminished glycemic reserve[9,51,52]. A retrospective study by Jensen et al. [53] showed that infants with gastroschisis who received cycled PN were approximately one-third less likely to develop IFALD compared with infants who received continuous PN.

Histopathological Changes

The histopathological changes of IF-associated cholestasis present a spectrum from hepatic steatosis to biliary cirrhosis [4]. Hepatic steatosis is more common in adults and may develop without evidence of inflammation, cholestasis, or hepatocyte necrosis [4,54]. Hepatic steatosis is less common in infants who are more likely to present with centrilobular cholestasis, portal inflammation, and necrosis with or without fatty infiltration [4]. More advanced liver disease has been described in children who are being evaluated for combined liver and small bowel transplantation and include portal fibrosis (100%), pericellular fibrosis (95%), and bile ductular proliferation (90%). Pigmented Kupffer cells (81%) and portal bridging (86%) were also prominent features. Cholestasis is not always present [4].

Table 2. Intestinal Failure–Associated Liver Disease Prevention and Treatment based on Pathophysiology (Adapted from Sukhotnik)

Pathophysiology	Suggested treatment
Disruption of enterohepatic cycle (ileal resection).	Encourage enteral feeding Stimulate the enterobiliary axis by breast milk, long-chain triglycerides or cholecystokinin analogs injection.
Inadequate macronutrient intake such as continuous PN infusion with excessive glucose intake and inadequate amino acid supply.	Encourage enteral feeding Reduce duration/adapt PN Use newly pediatric adapted amino acid solutions. Perform cyclic PN
Excessive intake of long-chain polyunsaturated fatty acids (PUFAs) with subsequent lipoperoxidation and high content of phytosterols from soybean oil–based emulsions.	Limit daily administration of intravenous lipids to 2–2.5 g/kg. Use newly fish oil based lipid solutions Stop intravenous lipids as soon as thrombocytopenia, hyperbilirubinemia, and/or jaundice appear.
Increased omega-6/omega-3 PUFA ratio.	Increase use of a fish oil-based intravenous lipid emulsions
Aluminium, iron, or chromium overload	Adapt iron intake and decrease PN solution aluminium content.
Intestinal stasis with subsequent intraluminal bacterial overgrowth with translocation (endotoxinemia) and/or release of inducible pro-inflammatory mediators (such as TNF)	Reduce bacterial overgrowth by antibiotics and/or performing tapering enteroplasty.
Recurrent catheter-related sepsis.	Central line care Multidisciplinary aseptic approach
Direct hepatotoxicity due to the hepatic immaturity in disposing potentially toxic substances.	Oral decontamination/probiotics fiber/glutamine Ursodeoxycholic acid 15–20 mg/k

Hepatic Steatosis

Hepatic steatosis is associated with hepatic accumulation of lipid or glycogen from excess calories (8–12 mg/kg/d of glucose) [4,55]. It is thought that parenteral carbohydrate calories are converted to triglyceride, perhaps by stimulating insulin release or by lipogenesis and the sythesis of acylglycerol from glucose as shown in rats [56]. Histology of the liver reveals fatty infiltration of hepatocytes, which is reversible after reduction of calories [54]. Hepatitic steatosis may also be related to excess lipid infusions; deficiencies of essential fatty acids; choline, taurine, or glutathione; or photoxidation of parenteral vitamins as shown in rats [4].

Feeding beyond the liver's ability to utilize carbohydrate and fat can cause accumulation of by-products in the liver and thereby result in IFALD. IFALD is potentially reversible if enteral feeding can be resumed and the TPN discontinued before the development of severe fibrosis or cirrhosis [4,57]. In many children and adults, this is not possible and prevention or treatment of IFALD includes a number of approaches listed in table 2 although not all have been proven to be successful [4].

Liver/Intestinal Transplantation

Patients with liver and intestinal failure who are not predicted to achieve intestinal rehabilitation and for whom death is otherwise unavoidable should be offered a combined liver and intestinal transplant [9]. Isolated liver transplant may be a successful strategy for select infants with SBS and IFALD in whom the residual bowel has the potential for intestinal adaptation [9]. It is believed that significant liver disease may hamper intestinal adaptation, and, thus, an isolated liver transplant may allow for more complete intestinal adaptation [58].

Accurately identifying children who have the potential for bowel adaptation remains difficult, and although there is no set of definitive criteria, important considerations include bowel length and maximal enteral tolerance [59,60]. Although an isolated liver transplant may be an option for some children, the outcome of an isolated liver transplant in a child with IFALD is dismal, having a 3-year survival of only 64% [61]. In addition, there is no protective effect of a mature donor liver on the recurrence of IFALD.

Prevention of IFALD

Preventative strategies are the cornerstone of improving outcomes in IFALD and include institution of enteral feedings, early weaning and cycling of PN, reduction in the dose of lipid emulsions administered with PN and strongly consider fish oil–based lipid emulsions. Early recognition, aggressive treatment, and prevention of sepsis are part of the measures that should be employed. Although there may be a role for surgical intervention, the risks and benefits involving the exact timing and nature of the surgical procedure must be carefully considered. While transplantation remains an option for children with end-stage liver disease, it is still associated with significant morbidity and mortality [9].

Early Institution of Enteral Feeds

Even minimal EN, often referred to as trophic feeding or gut-priming, promotes human intestinal epithelial cell growth and brush border enzyme activity and motility [9,62]. Enteral feeding, when administered continuously, can promote saturation of the intestinal transporters, thereby maximizing gut absorption [9,63] while gradually increasing enteral tolerance and advancement of feeds. Studies have shown that EN, when tolerated, may help to protect against the development of IFALD [9,64,65].

Enteral Type and Route

The type and route of EN can influence duration and success of weaning PN. The use of breast milk (BM) has been shown to correlate with shorter PN courses and to promote intestinal adaptation. [9,15,66]. Beneficial components of BM include high levels of nucleotides, amino acids, and immunologic and growth factors [9]. BM also has anti-infectious properties, and glycoproteins in BM deliver iron to the intestinal epithelium, stimulate proliferation and differentiation of crypt cells, influence brush border enzyme activity, and function as scavengers to prevent free radical–mediated tissue damage9. There are only a few studies investigating the role of breast milk in decreasing IFALD. Kulkarni et al. [67] conducted a retrospective analysis of newborns requiring prolonged parenteral nutrition. They divided the sample into three different groups (exclusive breast feeding, exclusive formula feeding and mixed feeding). Baseline characteristics, feeding profiles, liver enzymes and liver function tests were compared amongst the three groups. They found that among infants on PN for greater than 4 weeks, those who were exclusively breast fed were significantly less likely to develop IFALD [34.6%] compared to those who were only fed formula milk (72.7%).The mean maximum conjugated bilirubin and the mean maximum AST were significantly lower in the breast fed group compared to the formula fed group. Aside from BM, amino acid–based formulas, have similarly been associated with a shorter duration of PN-dependence [9,15,68,69]. Proposed explanations for improved outcomes with these formulas include a reduced incidence of food allergy and a high percentage of long-chain triglycerides (LCT), which have been shown to stimulate mucosal adaptation better than medium-chain triglycerides (MCT) [9,68,70,71].

Ursodeoxycholic Acid

Ursodeoxycholic acid (Ursodiol), a dihydroxy bile acid and choleretic agent developed according to the structure of bile in Chinese black bears, functions to improve bile flow and reduce the formation of biliary sludge, and has been widely used in various chronic cholestatic conditions [9]. This drug may be helpful in correcting the liver biochemical abnormalities seen with prolonged PN use in humans; however, the data available to date on the efficacy of this drug for neonates and children with IFALD remain inconclusive. Spagnuolo et al. [72] conducted an initial pilot study and found disappearance of cholestatic liver disease signs and normalization of biochemical markers of cholestasis within 4 to 8 weeks in 7 children receiving long term PN treated with Ursodiol. Two subsequent retrospective reports supported this conclusion and found that treatment with Ursodiol led to an early sustained decrease in serum bilirubin levels after 2 weeks of therapy in premature infants [73], reduced the duration of cholestasis, and decreased the peak conjugated bilirubin in very low birth weight infants with IFALD [74].

The most important contribution to the prevention and treatment of liver diseases is provided by intestinal rehabilitation that allows intravenous intake of glucose and lipids to be reduced below the relatively safe boundary of 7 or 1 g/kg bodyweight respectively [5]. A British study of adults with IF showed that cooperation between centers and local hospitals in performing home parenteral nutrition can reduce the complication rate to a lower level [75]. Experience from Canada shows that the treatment of patients in a pediatric short bowel syndrome center based on clear guidelines on parenteral nutrition, swift weaning off parenteral feeding, and aggressive treatment of complications reduces the incidence of liver diseases and increases the survival rate [76].

Conclusion

The occurrence of IFALD needs to be markedly reduced by appropriate early management, including surgical procedures aiming at preservation of as much bowel as possible as well as of the ileocoecal valve, and at primary bowel anastomosis, meticulous hygiene for prevention of early infections, and optimal professional management of parenteral nutrition. The potential benefits of providing fish oils for both treatment and prevention of IFALD are supported by plausible hypotheses and experimental data [17]. However, at this time, no controlled trials are available that would allow final conclusions on efficacy and safety and concerns remain with regards to potential untoward effects of prolonged intravenous administration of an emulsion based only on fish oil [17].

References

[1] O'Keefe SJ, Buchman AL, Fishbein TM, Jeejeebhoy KN, Jeppesen PB, Shaffer J. Short bowel syndrome and intestinal failure: consensus definitions and overview. *Clin Gastroenterol Hepatol.* 2006;4:6-10.

[2] Le HD, Fallon EM, de Meijer VE, Malkan AD, Puder M, Gura KM. Innovative parenteral and enteral nutrition therapy for intestinal failure. *Semin Pediatr Surg.* 2010;19:27-34.

[3] Squires RH, Duggan C, Teitelbaum DH, Wales PW, Balint J, Venick R, et al. Natural history of pediatric intestinal failure: initial report from the pediatric intestinal failure consortium. *J Pediatr.* 2012;161:723-728.

[4] Kelly DA. Intestinal failure-associated liver disease: what do we know today? Gastroenterology. 2006;130:S70-S77.

[5] Lloyd DA, Gabe SM. Managing liver dysfunction in parenteral nutrition. *Proc Nutr Soc.* 2007;66:530-538.

[6] Ching YA, Gura K, Modi B, Jaksic T. Pediatric intestinal failure: nutrition, pharmacologic, and surgical approaches. *Nutr Clin Pract.* 2007;22:653-663.

[7] Mazariegos GV, Squires RH, Sindhi RK. Current perspectives on pediatric intestinal transplantation. *Curr Gastroenterol Rep.* 2009;11:226-233.

[8] Squires RH, Duggan C, Teitelbaum DH, Wales PW, Balint J, Venick R, et al. Natural history of pediatric intestinal failure: initial report from the Pediatric Intestinal Failure Consortium. *J Pediatr.* 2012;161:723-728.

[9] Nehra D, Fallon EM, Puder M. The prevention and treatment of intestinal failure-associated liver disease in neonates and children. *Surg Clin North Am.* 2011;91:543-563.

[10] Kaufman SS, Pehlivanova M, Fennelly EM, Rekhtman YM, Gondolesi GE, Little CA, et al. Predicting liver failure in parenteral nutrition-dependent short bowel syndrome of infancy. *J Pediatr.* 2010;156:580-585.

[11] Diaz JJ, Gura KM, Roda J, Perez-Atayde AR ,Duggan C, Jaksic T, et al. AST to Platelet Index Correlates with Hepatic Cirrhosis But Not with Fibrosis in Pediatric Patients with Intestinal Failure. *J Pediatr Gastroenterol Nutr.* 2013.

[12] Quiros-Tejeira RE, Ament ME, Reyen L, Herzog F, Merjanian M , Olivares-Serrano N, et al. Long-term parenteral nutritional support and intestinal adaptation in children with short bowel syndrome: a 25-year experience. *J Pediatr.* 2004;145:157-163.

[13] Willis TC, Carter BA, Rogers SP, Hawthorne KM, Hicks PD, Abrams SA. High rates of mortality and morbidity occur in infants with parenteral nutrition-associated cholestasis. *JPEN J Parenter Enteral Nutr.* 2010;34:32-37.

[14] Chan S, McCowen KC, Bistrian BR, Thibault A, Keane-Ellison M, Forse RA, et al. Incidence, prognosis, and etiology of end-stage liver disease in patients receiving home total parenteral nutrition. *Surgery.* 1999;126:28-34.

[15] Andorsky DJ, Lund DP, Lillehei CW, Jaksic T, Dicanzio J, Richardson DS, et al. Nutritional and other postoperative management of neonates with short bowel syndrome correlates with clinical outcomes. *J Pediatr.* 2001;139:27-33.

[16] Diamanti A, Basso MS, Castro M, Calce A, Pietrobattista A, Gambarara M. Prevalence of life-threatening complications in pediatric patients affected by intestinal failure. *Transplant Proc.* 2007;39:1632-1633.

[17] Koletzko B, Goulet O. oil containing intravenous lipid emulsions in parenteral nutrition-associated cholestatic liver disease. *Curr Opin Clin Nutr Metab Care.* 2010;13:321-326.

[18] Hsieh MH, Pai W, Tseng HI, Yang SN, Lu CC, Chen HL. Parenteral nutrition-associated cholestasis in premature babies: risk factors and predictors. *Pediatr Neonatol.* 2009;50:202-207.

[19] Robinson DT, Ehrenkranz RA. Parenteral nutrition-associated cholestasis in small for gestational age infants. *J Pediatr.* 2008;152: 59-62.

[20] Greenberg GR, Wolman SL, Christofides ND, Bloom SR, Jeejeebhoy KN. Effect of total parenteral nutrition on gut hormone release in humans. *Gastroenterology.* 1981;80:988-993.

[21] Shulman RJ. New developments in total parenteral nutrition for children. *Curr Gastroenterol Rep.* 2000;2:253-258.

[22] Lucas A, Bloom SR, Aynsley-Green A. Gut hormones and 'minimal enteral feeding'. *Acta Paediatr Scand.* 1986;75:719-723.

[23] Jawaheer G, Pierro A, Lloyd DA, Shaw NJ. Gall bladder contractility in neonates: effects of parenteral and enteral feeding. *Arch Dis Child Fetal Neonatal Ed.* 1995;72:F200-F202.

[24] Bishay M, Pichler J, Horn V, Macdonald S, Ellmer M, Eaton S, et al. Intestinal failure-associated liver disease in surgical infants requiring long-term parenteral nutrition. *J Pediatr Surg.* 2012;47:359-362.

[25] Pichler J, Horn V, Macdonald S, Hill S. Intestinal failure-associated liver disease in hospitalised children. *Arch Dis Child.* 2012;9.214-7:211

[26] Beale EF, Nelson RM, Bucciarelli RL, Donnelly WH, Eitzman DV. Intrahepatic cholestasis associated with parenteral nutrition in premature infants. *Pediatrics.* 1979;64:342-347.

[27] Beath SV, Davies P, Papadopoulou A, Khan AR, Buick RG, Corkery JJ, et al. Parenteral nutrition-related cholestasis in postsurgical neonates: multivariate analysis of risk factors. *J Pediatr Surg.* 1996;31:604-606.

[28] Drongowski RA, Coran AG. An analysis of factors contributing to the development of total parenteral nutrition-induced cholestasis. *JPEN J Parenter Enteral Nutr.* 1989;13:586-589.

[29] O'Keefe SJ. Bacterial overgrowth and liver complications in short bowel intestinal failure patients. *Gastroenterology.* 2006;130:S67-S69.

[30] Goulet O, Joly F, Corriol O, Colomb-Jung V. Some new insights in intestinal failure-associated liver disease. *Curr Opin Organ Transplant.* 2009;14:256-261.

[31] Nordenstrom J, Jarstrand C, Wiernik A. Decreased chemotactic and random migration of leukocytes during Intralipid infusion. *Am J Clin Nutr.* 1979;32:2416-2422.

[32] Colomb V, Jobert-Giraud A, Lacaille F, Goulet O, Fournet JC, Ricour C. Role of lipid emulsions in cholestasis associated with long-term parenteral nutrition in children. *JPEN J Parenter Enteral Nutr.* 2000.350-24:345;

[33] Alwayn IP, Gura K, Nose V, Zausche B, Javid P, Garza J, et al. Omega-3 fatty acid supplementation prevents hepatic steatosis in a murine model of nonalcoholic fatty liver disease. *Pediatr Res.* 2005;57:445-452.

[34] Gura KM, Duggan CP, Collier SB, Jennings RW, Folkman J, Bistrian BR, et al. Reversal of parenteral nutrition-associated liver disease in two infants with short bowel syndrome using parenteral fish oil: implications for future management. *Pediatrics.* 2006;118:e197-e201.

[35] Puder M, Valim C, Meisel JA, Le HD, de Meijer VE, Robinson EM, et al. Parenteral fish oil improves outcomes in patients with parenteral nutrition-associated liver injury. *Ann Surg.* 2009;250:395-402.

[36] Diamond IR, Sterescu A, Pencharz PB, Wales PW. The rationale for the use of parenteral omega-3 lipids in children with short bowel syndrome and liver disease. *Pediatr Surg Int.* 2008;24:773-778.

[37] Tomsits E, Pataki M, Tolgyesi A, Fekete G, Rischak K, Szollar L. Safety and efficacy of a lipid emulsion containing a mixture of soybean oil, medium-chain triglycerides, olive oil, and fish oil: a randomised, double-blind clinical trial in premature infants requiring parenteral nutrition. *J Pediatr Gastroenterol Nutr.* 2010;51:514-521.

[38] Mertes N, Grimm H ,Furst P, Stehle P. Safety and efficacy of a new parenteral lipid emulsion (SMOFlipid) in surgical patients: a randomized, double-blind, multicenter study. *Ann Nutr Metab.* 2006;50:253-259.

[39] Mirtallo J, Canada T, Johnson D, Kumpf V, Petersen C, Sacks G, et al. Safe practices for parenteral nutrition. *JPEN J Parenter Enteral Nutr.* 2004;28:S39-S70.

[40] Wessel JJ, Kocoshis SA. Nutritional management of infants with short bowel syndrome. *Semin Perinatol.* 2007;31:104-111.

[41] Cavicchi M, Beau P, Crenn P, Degott C, Messing B. Prevalence of liver disease and contributing factors in patients receiving home parenteral nutrition for permanent intestinal failure. *Ann Intern Med.* 2000;132:525-532.

[42] Crawford MA, Costeloe K, Ghebremeskel K, Phylactos A. The inadequacy of the essential fatty acid content of present preterm feeds. *Eur J Pediatr.* 1998;157 Suppl 1:S23-S27.

[43] Innis SM. Omega-3 Fatty acids and neural development to 2 years of age: do we know enough for dietary recommendations? *J Pediatr Gastroenterol Nutr.* 2009;48 Suppl 1:S16-S24.

[44] Rigo J, Senterre J. Is taurine essential for the neonates? *Biol Neonate.* 1977;32:73-76.

[45] Cooke RJ, Whitington PF, Kelts D. Effect of taurine supplementation on hepatic function during short-term parenteral nutrition in the premature infant. *J Pediatr Gastroenterol Nutr.* 1984;3:234-238.

[46] von RH, Hannman T, Subotic U, Brade J, Schaible T, Waag KL, et al. Use of di(2-ethylhexyl)phthalate-containing infusion systems increases the risk for cholesta. *Pediatrics.* 2009;124:710-716.

[47] Bohrer D, do Nascimento PC, Binotto R, Becker E, Pomblum S. Contribution of the raw material to the aluminum contamination in parenterals. *JPEN J Parenter Enteral Nutr.* 2002;26:382-388.

[48] Bougle D, Bureau F, Deschrevel G, Hecquard C, Neuville D, Drosdowsky M, et al. Chromium and parenteral nutrition in children. *J Pediatr Gastroenterol Nutr.* 1993;17:72-74.

[49] Fell JM, Reynolds AP, Meadows N, Khan K, Long SG, Quaghebeur G, et al. Manganese toxicity in children receiving long-term parenteral nutrition. *Lancet.* 1996;347:1218-1221.

[50] Reynolds AP, Kiely E, Meadows N. Manganese in long term paediatric parenteral nutrition. *Arch Dis Child.* 1994;71:527-528.

[51] Collier S, Crough J, Hendricks K, Caballero B. Use of cyclic parenteral nutrition in infants less than 6 months of age. *Nutr Clin Pract.* 1994;9:65-68.

[52] Takehara H, Hino M, Kameoka K, Komi N. A new method of total parenteral nutrition for surgical neonates: it is possible that cyclic TPN prevents intrahepatic cholestasis. *Tokushima J Exp Med.* 1990;37:97-102.

[53] Jensen AR, Goldin AB, Koopmeiners JS, Stevens J, Waldhausen JH, Kim SS. The association of cyclic parenteral nutrition and decreased incidence of cholestatic liver disease in patients with gastroschisis. *J Pediatr Surg.* 2009;44:183-189.

[54] Tulikoura I, Huikuri K. Morphological fatty changes and function of the liver, serum free fatty acids, and triglycerides during parenteral nutrition. *Scand J Gastroenterol.* 1982;17:177-185.

[55] Zaman N ,Tam YK, Jewell LD, Coutts RT. Effects of intravenous lipid as a source of energy in parenteral nutrition associated hepatic dysfunction and lidocaine elimination: a study using isolated rat liver perfusion. *Biopharm Drug Dispos.* 1997;18:803-819.

[56] Meguid MM, Chen TY, Yang ZJ, Campos AC, Hitch DC, Gleason JR. Effects of continuous graded total parenteral nutrition on feeding indexes and metabolic concomitants in rats. *Am J Physiol.* 1991;260:E126-E140.

[57] Dahms BB, Halpin TC, Jr. Serial liver biopsies in parenteral nutrition-associated cholestasis of early infancy. *Gastroenterology.* 1981;81:136-144.

[58] Goulet O, Kamin D. Intestinal failure, short bowel syndrome, and intestinal transplantation. In: Duggan C, Watkins JB, Walker WA, editors. *Nutrition in pediatrics.* 4th ed. BC Decker; 2007. 641-662.

[59] Horslen SP, Sudan DL, Iyer KR, Kaufman SS, Iverson AK, Fox IJ, et al. Isolated liver transplantation in infants with end-stage liver disease associated with short bowel syndrome. *Ann Surg.* 2002;235: 435-439.

[60] Botha JF, Grant WJ, Torres C, Iverson AK, Sudan DL, Shaw BW, Jr., et al. Isolated liver transplantation in infants with end-stage liver disease due to short bowel syndrome. *Liver Transpl.* 2006;12:1062-1066.

[61] Dell-Olio D, Beath SV, de Ville de GJ, Clarke S, Davies P, Lloyd C, et al. Isolated liver transplant in infants with short bowel syndrome: insights into outcomes and prognostic factors. *J Pediatr Gastroenterol Nutr.* 2009;48:334-340.

[62] Perdikis DA, Basson MD. Basal nutrition promotes human intestinal epithelial (Caco-2) proliferation, brush border enzyme activity, and motility. *Crit Care Med.* 1997;25:159-165.

[63] Parker P, Stroop S, Greene H. A controlled comparison of continuous versus intermittent feeding in the treatment of infants with intestinal disease. *J Pediatr.* 1981;99:360-364.

[64] Zamir O, Nussbaum MS, Bhadra S, Subbiah MT, Rafferty JF, Fischer JE. Effect of enteral feeding on hepatic steatosis induced by total parenteral nutrition. *JPEN J Parenter Enteral Nutr.* 1994; 18: 20-25.

[65] Meehan JJ, Georgeson KE. Prevention of liver failure in parenteral nutrition-dependent children with short bowel syndrome. *J Pediatr Surg.* 1997;32:473-475.

[66] Playford RJ, Macdonald CE, Johnson WS. Colostrum and milk-derived peptide growth factors for the treatment of gastrointestinal disorders. *Am J Clin Nutr.* 2000;72:5-14.

[67] Kulkarni S, Mercado V, Rios M, Arboleda R, Gomara R, Muinos W, et al. Breast Milk is Better Than Formula Milk in Preventing Parenteral Nutrition Associated Liver Disease [PNALD] in Infants on Prolonged Parenteral Nutrition. *J Pediatr Gastroenterol Nutr.* 2013.

[68] Vanderhoof JA. New and emerging therapies for short bowel syndrome in children. *J Pediatr Gastroenterol Nutr.* 2004;39 Suppl 3:S769-S771.

[69] Bines J, Francis D, Hill D. Reducing parenteral requirement in children with short bowel syndrome: impact of an amino acid-based complete infant formula. *J Pediatr Gastroenterol Nutr.* 1998;26:123-128.

[70] Vanderhoof JA, Grandjean CJ, Kaufman SS, Burkley KT, Antonson DL. Effect of high percentage medium-chain triglyceride diet on mucosal adaptation following massive bowel resection in rats. *JPEN J Parenter Enteral Nutr.* 1984;8:685-689.

[71] Kollman KA, Lien EL, Vanderhoof JA. Dietary lipids influence intestinal adaptation after massive bowel resection. *J Pediatr Gastroenterol Nutr.* 1999;28:41-45.

[72] Spagnuolo MI, Iorio R, Vegnente A, Guarino A. Ursodeoxycholic acid for treatment of cholestasis in children on long-term total parenteral nutrition: a pilot study. *Gastroenterology.* 1996;111:716-719.

[73] Levine A, Maayan A, Shamir R, Dinari G, Sulkes J, Sirotta L. Parenteral nutrition-associated cholestasis in preterm neonates: evaluation of ursodeoxycholic acid treatment. *J Pediatr Endocrinol Metab.* 1999; 12: 549-553.

[74] Chen CY, Tsao PN, Chen HL, Chou HC, Hsieh WS, Chang MH. Ursodeoxycholic acid (UDCA) therapy in very-low-birth-weight infants with parenteral nutrition-associated cholestasis. *J Pediatr.* 2004;145:317-321.

[75] Freshwater DA, Saadeddin A, Deel-Smith P, Digger T, Jones BJ. Can home parenteral nutrition be provided by non-specialised centres? 2300 weeks of experience at a district general hospital in the United Kingdom. *Clin Nutr.* 2005;24:229-235.

[76] Sigalet D, Boctor D, Robertson M ,Lam V, Brindle M, Sarkhosh K, et al. Improved outcomes in paediatric intestinal failure with aggressive prevention of liver disease. *Eur J Pediatr Surg.* 2009;19:348-353.

In: Short Bowel Syndrome in Children
Editor: Igor Sukhotnik
ISBN: 978-1-62948-518-8

Chapter VI

Management of Short Bowel Syndrome

Rima Sohotnik and Ori Segol, M.D.
Department of Gastroenterology, Carmel Medical Center,
Technion-Israel Institute of Technology,
The Ruth & Bruce Rappaport Faculty of Medicine, Haifa, Israel

Abstract

Management of children after massive bowel resection is optimized by interdisciplinary coordination of parenteral and enteral nutrition support, medical management of associated complications, surgical lengthening procedures, and intestinal transplantation. Individual plans of care are developed based on the length and sites of remaining bowel, the degree of intestinal adaptation, and the patient's ability to adhere to the medication and dietary regimens. Although patients require parenteral nutrition and/or intravenous fluids in the immediate postresection period, diet and enteral nutrition should be reintroduced as soon as possible. Antisecretory and antidiarrheal medications are prescribed to slow intestinal transit times and optimize fluid and nutrient absorption. The purpose of this chapter is to discuss the newest methods of optimizing pediatric parenteral and enteral nutrition in patients with SBS while ensuring growth, promoting intestinal adaptation, and reducing associated complications.

Keywords: Short bowel syndrome, intestinal failure, bowel resection, management, total parenteral nutrition, intestinal associated liver disease, SMOFlipid, omegaven, enteral nutrition, fat-soluble vitamins, water-soluble vitamins, zinc, manganese, selenium, antidiarrheal agent, antisecretory agent, pancreatic enzymes, antimicrobials, teduglutide

Introduction

Management of short bowel syndrome (SBS) primarily focuses on intestinal rehabilitation using a multidisciplinary approach including nutritional, medical and surgical interventions to improve the function of the remnant small intestine and achieve the goal of full enteral nutrition [1-3]. Supplemental parenteral support (PS; parenteral nutrition and/or intravenous [PN/IV] fluids) is required to maintain fluid, electrolytes, trace elements, vitamins, and nutrient balances in patients with SBS with intestinal failure (SBS-IF). Treatments aim to maximize remnant intestinal absorptive capacity, to minimize the symptoms of malabsorption, to minimize, avoid or eliminate the need for PS. Management of SBS has traditionally been divided into three phases: an acute phase, an adaptation phase, and a maintenance phase. The first stage of care begins after resuscitation of the patient in the post-operative period or at the time the diagnosis of short bowel syndrome has been made [4]. This phase is marked by poor absorption of almost all nutrients, including water, electrolytes, proteins, carbohydrates, fats, vitamins, and trace elements [5]. Fluid loss from the gastrointestinal tract tends to be greatest during the first few days after massive small intestinal resection. Aggressive fluid and electrolyte replacement therapy is necessary to reduce life-threatening dehydration, hypotension, and electrolyte imbalances. During this time a permanent silastic central venous catheter needs to be inserted. Since the child will need long-term venous access, each access site must be carefully cared for and protected. The child's main or sole caloric source will be via the parenteral route for a considerable period of time. Nevertheless, enteral feedings should be initiated within 1 to 2 weeks after the onset of the short-bowel syndrome. Scolapio and Fleming described therapeutic guidelines for the fluid and electrolyte management of these patients [6]. These include replacement of fluid and electrolytes lost through nasogastric suctioning and in stool. They recommended that 300-500mL be added to the total volume administered to replace insensible losses. These replacement volumes are added to the patient's calculated daily maintenance volume. Daily urine output should be at least 1 L. Phase II, the adaptation phase, generally begins within 24 to 48 hours after resection and may last from 1 to 2 years [7]. During the second phase of support, a more stabilized state has been reached, at which point careful monitoring of the patient's nutritional status is very important. Electrolytes, liver function tests and assessment of protein status (total protein, albumin and total iron-binding capacity) should be done initially and on a weekly basis. Fat-soluble vitamin levels should be assessed approximately every six months to assure that adequate amounts are being absorbed. Serum levels of vitamins A, D and E can be assayed. A prothrombin time will be indicative of vitamin K levels. Patients with a significant loss of the terminal ileum should have a vitamin B12 level assessed on a yearly basis. Supplementation of fat-soluble vitamins, if depleted, should also be carried out. During this period, 90% to 95% of the bowel adaptation potential (including nutritional and metabolic stability) has been realized, and only 5% to 10% of additional improvement in bowel adaptation and absorption is possible [4]. Adaptive changes also take place in the stomach, pancreas, and colon. Clinical manifestations of intestinal adaptation include weight change and stabilization of fluid and electrolyte levels [8]. Carbonnel and others wrote that little bowel compensation occurs after 3 months [9]. Data from animal studies conducted by Wilmore and colleagues suggested that supplementing enteral intake with parenteral nutrition early in the postoperative course results in better overall bowel adaptation. [10]. This is most likely because it facilitates provision of adequate calorie and nitrogen sources. According to Nightingale and colleagues, when enteral nutrient absorption falls to below one third of premorbid capacity, some amount of parenteral nutrition is needed [11]. Parenteral nutrition can be started with standard formulations and administered over the course of 24 hours daily on an inpatient basis. Make efforts to infuse daily requirements in shorter time periods before the patient is discharged. This is called cycling and it allows liberation from the solution pump for at least some time each day. In addition, laboratory studies, including serum chemistries and mineral and trace element levels, are monitored frequently and provision of these nutrients adjusted accordingly in the parenteral nutrition formula. Gradually, most patients are able to resume and increase oral food intake. This is begun by providing small frequent feedings and slowly advancing the diet as tolerated. According to Scolapio and Fleming, the process of weaning the patient off parenteral nutrition can begin once oral calorie intake exceeds 1000 kcal/d [12]. Further reductions in parenteral nutrition are predicated on increased oral intake. Woolf and associates reported that nutrient absorption is not complete in patients with loss of half or more of the small bowel [13]. Therefore, they usually require 30-40 kcal/kg/d to meet daily energy requirements.

By phase III, the maintenance phase, the absorptive capacity of the gut is at a maximum leading the patient to wean from parenteral nutrition. During this stage, which may last from months to years, a variety of factors must also be monitored. These include an assurance that the child will develop normal suck and swallow reflexes and not develop an aversion to oral feedings. Also, the child should be monitored for normal length and weight gain. Finally, patients with an intact colon should be evaluated for the development of renal oxalate stones, and, thus, should avoid a high oxalate diet. Attempts should be made to compensate for continued malabsorption by increasing the quantity of small meals and supplementation with vitamins and minerals. At this point, the patient has either adapted maximally so that nutritional and metabolic homeostasis can be achieved entirely by oral feeding, or the patient is committed to receiving supplemental or complete nutritional support for life, either by ambulatory home TPN and/or specialized enteral or oral feedings. Prebiotic or probiotic therapy may be beneficial for patients with SBS, although further research is needed to determine optimal protocols. Patients with SBS, particularly those without a colon, are at high risk of dehydration; oral rehydration solutions sipped throughout the day can help maintain hydration. One of the primary goals of SBS therapy is to reduce or eliminate dependence on PN/IV; optimization of EN and hydration substantially increases the probability of successful PN/IV weaning [14].

A. Assessment of Nutritional and Fluid Status

In the immediate postoperative period, all patients will require intravenous fluids and electrolytes to replace losses. Fluid and electrolyte management is the most critical part of medical management for the patient with SBS. Virtually no patient with this disorder requires macronutrient supplementation alone, but patients may often be weaned successfully from TPN, yet still require fluid and electrolyte support. During the initial 6 months after massive enterectomy, gastric hypersecretion develops [15] Basal acid secretion as well as gastrin secretion significantly increase. These increases are associated with an increased risk for peptic ulcer disease as well as with increased fluid losses. In addition, at an acidic pH, pancreatic lipase is deactivated and fat maldigestion worsens. Therefore, high-dose intravenous H_2 receptor antagonists or oral proton-pump inhibitors should be prescribed during this period. Just as nutrient malabsorption occurs, so does medication malabsorption, and therefore, increased doses of orally administered medication may be required. Fluid losses can be controlled with antimotility agents, such as loperamide hydrochloride or diphenoxylate (4-16 mg/day). Patients whose fluid losses are not controlled and who develop dehydration may require codeine (15-60 mg, 3-4 times daily) or a tincture of opium. Rarely, patients with proximal jejunostomy and several liters of daily stomal output will require octreotide (50-100 mcg sc, 2-4 times daily) [16]. Its use should be discouraged because animal studies have suggested that octreotide inhibits intestinal adaptation and increases the risk for cholelithiasis.

Oral rehydration solutions (ORS) are important in the maintenance of adequate fluid balance and help decrease the need for parenteral fluids - this is especially critical in patients with proximal jejunostomies who are net fluid and sodium excretors. The jejunum is permeable to sodium and chloride; therefore, solutions with a high NaCl content are readily and passively absorbed. Neither sodium nor water is absorbed from hypo- or isotonic solutions in the jejunum. In addition, glucose promotes both salt and water absorption via "solvent drag." Sodium and glucose absorption are mediated by a cotransporter. Although ORS do not decrease fluid losses, their use increases intracellular hydration. Several commercial formulas are available, although the least costly option is for the patient to formulate the solution recommended by the World Health Organization at home. The patient is instructed to mix 2.5 g of NaCl (table salt), 20 g of glucose (table sugar), 1.5 g of KCl (requires prescription), and 2.5 g of Na_2CO_2 in 1 L of tap water [17]. The critical aspect of ORS is that the optimal sodium concentration should be in the range of 90-120 mEq/L [18]. Most commercially available solutions have substantially less sodium. The use of solutions with less sodium may result in increased sodium loss. Therefore, patients should be strongly encouraged to avoid "plain" water consumption when they are thirsty and to substitute ORS. The need for ORS is not as critical for patients with colon in continuity as long as there is sufficient sodium in the diet because the colon readily absorbs the ion, even against a strong electrochemical gradient [19]. In addition, because ileal water absorption is unaffected by glucose, the glucose concentration of the ORS in patients whose jejunum has been resected has less importance [20]. Significant quantities of magnesium are lost in jejunal and ileal effluent - thus, magnesium deficiency may occur. This deficiency often develops despite a normal serum concentration; therefore, a 24-hour urine magnesium measurement is often required [21]. Supplementation may be problematic because magnesium is a cathartic; parenteral supplementation may be required. Magnesium deficiency may also result in calcium deficiency because of impaired parathyroid hormone release. Patients with short bowel syndrome who do not receive TPN are generally in negative calcium balance [22]. and a supplement (800–1500 mg/day) should be prescribed.

Other commercially prepared oral solutions are available in over-the-counter premixed bottles and closely approximate the World Health Organization solution [23].

B. Innovative Parenteral Nutrition Therapy for Short Bowel Syndrome

Optimization of nutritional support is important in enhancing the rehabilitation of patients with the short bowel syndrome. If the total amount of small intestine remaining is 100 cm or less, total parenteral nutrition (TPN) is essential for survival. The prognosis of SBS has greatly improved during the past decades as a result of TPN [24]. TPN and home TPN remains the mainstay of therapy, independent of the nature of intestinal failure, which can be total or partial and permanent or temporary. TPN usually may be initiated on the second or third postoperative day, when the patient's cardiovascular and pulmonary functions have stabilized. The TPN should consist of a majority of calories from fat, followed by protein, and the remaining as carbohydrates. Vitamins, minerals, and trace elements should also be added accordingly. Long-term use of TPN, however, is associated with many complications, including central venous catheter infection and sepsis, vascular thrombosis, metabolic abnormalities, and organ dysfunction. The most serious complication, is TPN-associated liver disease, also called intestinal associated liver disease (IFALD),with a prevalence of 25–33% in neonates [25]. The etiology of IFALD remains to be elucidated. A total of 25% to 100% of patients receiving long-term TPN develop liver enzyme abnormalities, and end-stage liver disease may develop in 15% to 40% of these patients [26]. When long-term TPN is given with a modest amount of total energy and a minimal amount of intravenous fat, abnormal liver enzyme levels are common, but severe liver dysfunction is unusual. Excess carbohydrates (>50 kcal/kg) and excess fat (>1 g/kg daily) are associated with steatosis and cholestasis [27]. Several innovative and potentially effective TPN approaches have been proposed to delay and possibly prevent complications associated with TPN-administration. Cycling TPN involves the provision of total daily TPN volume in less than 24 hours in goal to disconnect patient from the intravenous line, improve visceral protein stores, and reduce the incidence of hyperinsulinemia [28-29]. Cycling TPN is recommended for patients who are expected to be on prolonged courses of PN (i.e. >30 days) and whose cardiac, renal and endocrine function can tolerate shifts in fluid and dextrose infusion rates. Patients should be metabolically stable on their goal solutions for several days before attempting to cycle TPN. In an attempt to avoid hyper- or hypoglycemia, the infusion rate is gradually increased over 1-2 hours at the beginning of the infusion and gradually decreased over the final hour of the infusion. In neonates, cycling should be limited to 6 hrs off TPN due to diminished glycemic reserves.

TPN is typically administered in conjunction with an intravenous lipid emulsion (ILE) to provide a caloric dense alternative to dextrose as a source of non-protein calories, and to supply essential omega-3 and omega-6 fatty acids for biologic membranes and the maintenance of immune function [30]. Until 2010, only FDA approved lipid emulsions in the United States were comprised of safflower oil, soybean oil (Intralipid®, Baxter Healthcare, Fresenius Kabi), or a combination of the two (Liposyn II ®, Hospira), which are all rich in omega-6 fatty acids. Today, other ILEs that are approved for use in US and Europe include SMOFLipid® (Fresenius Kabi) and Omegaven® (Fresenius Kabi). These formulations utilize the potential anti-inflammatory benefit of omega-3 fatty acids. Most of our dietary fat is derived from vegetable oils, particularly soy oil, which is rich in the n-6 fatty acid linoleic acid (18:2n-6, LA). LA is the precursor of arachidonic acid (20:4n-6, AA). Especially linseed oil, and to a less extent rapeseed oil and soy oil contain substantial amounts of the n-3 FA α-linolenic acid (18:3n-3, ALA). However, in humans the *in vivo* conversion of ALA to the n-3 polyunsaturated fatty acids (PUFAs) eicosapentaenoic acid (20:5n-3, EPA), and particularly docosahexaenoic acid (22:6n-3, DHA), is limited. Thus, fatty fish and n-3 PUFA supplements are important sources of the 'marine' n-3 PUFAs EPA and DHA. These long chain n-3 PUFAs decrease the production of pro-inflammatory eicosanoids and cytokines, directly by replacing AA in blood and tissues and inhibiting AA metabolism or indirectly by altering gene transcription [31-33]. The current Western diet with excessive n-6 FAs compared with n-3 FAs yields a high ratio of n-6 to n-3 FAs, especially AA to EPA, e.g. in the cell membrane phospholipids. The transition from a soybean- to a fish oil-based lipid formulation, such as the ω-3 parenteral lipid formulation (Omegaven), has shown a dramatic reversal of IFALD within the pediatric population [34-35].

In 1984, taurine deficiency was reported in three children with severe IFALD [36]. Since taurine plays a role in many functions in the liver such as osmoregulation, membrane stability and anti-oxidation, its deficiency can cause liver damage. This is of concern since neonates receiving long-term TPN can develop taurine deficiency [37].

Sepsis is a major risk factor in the development of IFALD of patients with SBS [38]. Patients with recurrent episodes of infection have a 30% increased chance of developing IFALD [39]. The source of infection could be catheter-related, bacterial translocation from intestinal stasis, permeability, or bacterial overgrowth. Prevention of catheter-related infection is crucial in preventing and reducing the severity of IFALD. Several methods of prevention of catheter-related infection have been shown to be effective in children with SBS. In the TPN dependent child with SBS, maintaining the integrity of the central venous catheter is essential. Incidence of catheter-related infection approaches 60% over the life span of the catheter [40]. The increased morbidity and mortality associated with catheter-related infection has led to the use of various antibiotic and ethanol lock techniques [41,42]. Anti-infective locks including vancomycin, ciprofloxacin, gentamicin, and amphotericin B have been studied for the prevention of catheter-related infections, with efficacy ranging between 30–100% [43]. A prospective study using combination lock therapy with vancomycin and gentamicin demonstrated a significant decrease in bacteremia and clinical sepsis rate [44]. Recently, attention has concentrated on ethanol locks and their effectiveness in decreasing the rate of catheter-related infections. An advantage of ethanol as compared to antibiotic locks includes an absence of resistance. Ethanol denatures proteins and is rapidly bactericidal and fungicidal [45]. A prospective pilot study in 2008 documented safety and potential efficacy of ethanol locks in treating central venous catheter-associated infections [46]. Randomized controlled trials have recently shown the positive effects of ethanol locks on the prevention of catheter associated bacteremia and subsequent sepsis in children with SBS and a history of multiple catheter-related bloodstream infections [47].

C. Innovative Enteral Nutrition Therapy for Short Bowel Syndrome

Although TPN is initially necessary, luminal nutrition is essential for complete adaptation and should be initiated as early as possible. Enteral feeding is preferred because it is more economical, easier, and safer than TPN. Enteral feeding is also more physiological and exposes the gastrointestinal tract to nutrient and hormonal stimuli, which are not present when the patient is not fed enterally. Luminal substrates and intraluminal nutrients are essential for development of intestinal adaptation and can protect against stress-induced gastropathy and gastrointestinal hemorrhage. Even with minimal enteral nutrition (e.g. trophic feeds), human intestinal epithelial cell growth, brush-border enzyme activity and motility are enhanced. Initiation of feeding is therefore recommended early in the postoperative period. In patients with SBS, successful implementation of enteral and parenteral nutrition can greatly enhance the intestinal rehabilitation process and the patient's quality of life. Enteral nutrients (e.g., glutamine, soluble fibers, pectin, and short chain fatty acids) act directly via contact with intestinal epithelium; they also act indirectly to stimulate the secretion of intestinal trophic hormones (e.g., growth hormone, epidermal growth factor, insulin-like growth factor I), pancreaticobiliary secretions and gut hormones such as enteroglucagon and gastrin [48]. Patients with very short bowel (<60 cm) and those who do not tolerate oral feeds small feedings of isotonic liquids and solid foods should be initiated with improvement of the patient's and should be further maintained on a defined-formula diet. This may be accomplished by constant infusion, starting with a diluted diet infused at approximately 25 mL/h. Both the concentration and rate should be increased commensurate with the patient's tolerance until a concentration of 100 to 125 mL/h is reached [49]. When the patient's fluid and electrolyte balance has stabilized, bowel sounds have returned, and there is less than 2 L/d of diarrhea, an elemental diet may be initiated [50]. Early continuous feedings with high-viscosity enteral diets tend to reduce duration of TPN therapy, allowing earlier removal of central venous catheters. Originally, elemental diets were favored for patients with SBS because they are more effectively absorbed and have lower osmolarity than polymeric formulas [51]. Elemental diets are very efficiently absorbed within the first 100 cm of jejunum. Polymeric diets are easily taken orally, are less hyperosmolar, and are much less expensive than elemental formulations. For these reasons, most clinicians tend to prescribe polymeric diets initially, providing elemental diets only to those patients who are unable to tolerate polymeric formulas. However, some researchers argue that there is no significant difference in caloric absorption, stomal output, or electrolyte losses among elemental, polymeric, and normal diets in patients with SBS [52]. Patients with high-output stomas (more than 2L/day) may benefit from an additional 5 to 10 g of soluble fiber per day, which can be obtained from over-the-counter fiber supplements.

Although enteral lipids contain the highest caloric density compared with other nutrients, long chain fats are least tolerated in short bowel syndrome. The etiology of lipid malabsorption in SBS is multifactorial and includes a decrease in absorptive surface area, a reduced bile acid pool, relative pancreatic insufficiency, motility disorders of the remaining gut and bacterial overgrowth. The colon absorbs short-chain (C2-C6) fatty acids, but not the long-chain (C14-C18) fatty acids usually found in dietary fat. Patients with a colon who consume a high-fat diet may experience increased diarrhea as a result of increased secretion of water and sodium secondary to maldigestion of fatty acids. These patients may benefit from a diet high in complex carbohydrates (50–60% of calories) and lower in fat (30% of calories) [53]. It is generally believed that low fat diet results in less diarrhea, less steatorrhea, and better absorption of nutrients and micronutrients. Both diarrhea and steatorrhea may be decreased if dietary fat is reduced from 90–100 g to 20–40 g per day [54]. Fecal fat excretion may be reduced also in patients with SBS by replacing long-chain fatty acids in the diet with medium-chain fatty acids. The water-soluble medium-chain fatty acids are absorbed directly in the large intestine in a manner similar to that of short chain fatty acids, even in patients with virtually no absorption of long-chain fat. Nordgaard et al [55], in a crossover trial, randomized 14 patients with short bowel syndrome (8 with an intact colon and 6 with jejunostomies and no functioning colon) to a diet high in carbohydrate or a diet high in fat. For patients without a colon, manipulating the diet did not significantly affect energy absorption, but the high-carbohydrate diet increased stool output by more than 700 mL vs the high-fat diet.

Insoluble fibers or bulk fibers (e.g., wheat, bran) are poorly digested in SBS patient and increase excretion of nitrogen, calcium, zinc, and iron as well as increase fecal fat. Therefore, they should be avoided. In contrast, soluble fibers (pectin, guar gum) that are fermented in the colon to produce short chain fatty acids without an increase in bulk may be of benefit because they delay gastric emptying by increasing intragastric viscosity. In SBS, pectin serves as a precursor for short chain fatty acids, which increase oxygen uptake in the colon, therefore maintaining gut integrity. In addition, the addition of pectin to enteral feeds leads to more rapid adaptive responses in both the small and large intestine [56]. Despite reduced protein absorption, most patients with SBS who maintain a stable weight with oral nutrition alone do not require protein supplementation because they have a positive nitrogen balance. If protein deficiency is suspected, patients may be given 80 to 100 g of dietary protein daily [57,58]. Both fat-soluble and water-soluble vitamins should be accounted for in the SBS diet [59]. Serum 25 (OH) vitamin D levels can be normalized by giving 50,000 IU of oral vitamin D every other day until normalization of the plasma levels occurs. Patients with osteoporosis should also receive 1,500 mg of elemental calcium per day along with one multivitamin. While the endocrine action of the active metabolite 1,25-dihydroxyvitamin D has been well characterized in relation to the maintenance of plasma calcium and phosphate homeostasis through regulation of intestinal absorption, recent research has focused on its autocrine and/or paracrine activities. Such activities have been best characterized in intestine, where VitD regulates cell differentiation and maturation. In a recent study, effect of Vit D on enterocyte turnover was evaluated in a rat model of SBS. This study has shown that dietary supplementation with Vit D stimulates enterocyte turnover, which correlates with up-regulated Vit D receptor expression in the remaining small intestine [60].

Magnesium supplements are extremely important in preventing formation of calcium oxalate kidney stones in patients with steatorrhea. The decline in urinary magnesium occurs before that of serum magnesium and is a more reliable indicator of magnesium deficiency. Furthermore, parenterally administered magnesium tends to decrease the likelihood of formation of calcium oxalate stones. Thus, attempts at replacing magnesium in patients with gut failure should be aimed at normalizing urinary magnesium levels [61]. Since magnesium salts given enterally increase diarrhea, soluble magnesium salts given as part of an oral rehydration solution may be better tolerated and absorbed than other magnesium complexes [62]. Vitamin A can be replaced by a water-soluble aqueous preparation of 5,000 IU/0.1 cc dropper, and vitamin E tablets can be replaced with a solution of 4,600 IU/5 cc dropper. Vitamin K can be replaced by a 5-mg oral supplement per day and titrated to the frequency required to maintain a normal prothrombin time [52]. Of the water-soluble vitamins, vitamin B12 is the one that may need to be replaced in those patients with greater than 60 cm of ileal resection. Normal stores may last for 2 to 4 years, but some patients may have had inadequate vitamin B12 use before surgery. Because the enterohepatic circulation accounts for 10μg/d, total malabsorption would require 300μg/mo for replacement. Therefore, a monthly injection of 1,000 μg of vitamin B12 is adequate replacement therapy. Other water-soluble vitamins usually can be maintained with a daily oral multivitamin. Zinc may be lost in stool, nasogastric aspirates, and fistulous drainage. In these cases, intravenous replacement usually is necessary to restore the zinc balance. In less severe cases, a multivitamin with zinc will provide approximately 22 mg of elemental zinc (compared with the recommended daily allowance of 15 mg). Loss of zinc is high in patients with large-volume gastrointestinal output. These patients require large doses of oral zinc supplements because of limited zinc absorption. Serum zinc may also be low because of low serum albumin, the major zinc-binding protein; this may not necessarily reflect zinc deficiency. Other supplements that may be needed include potassium, manganese, selenium, and glucose [49]. It is rare for SBS patients who are maintained on an oral regimen to need a potassium supplement. If low serum potassium occurs, the possibility of chronic sodium depletion with secondary hyperaldosteronism or magnesium deficiency should be considered [63,64]. The water-soluble vitamins and minerals (vitamin B-complex and C, calcium, iron, magnesium) are absorbed in the proximal small intestine, whereas magnesium diffuses passively throughout the entire small bowel [65]. In an effort to improve bowel rehabilitation, the amino acid glutamine, growth hormone and a diet optimized to enhance absorption have been administered to 300 patients with the short bowel syndrome. Initially about 60% of the patients were weaned from TPN and an additional 30% had reduced TPN requirements. At long-term follow up (2 years) 40% of the group remained off TPN, 40% had reduced TPN requirements and 20% had the same requirements [66].

D. Pharmacologic Therapy

Several drugs may be useful in the treatment of SBS, depending on the amount and location of the loss of absorptive capacity. Pharmacologic treatment of short bowel includes antidiarrheal (eg, loperamide hydrochloride, diphenoxylate and atropine, codeine, paregoric, and tincture of opium) and antisecretory agents (eg, histamine2-blockers, protonpump inhibitors, octreotide acetate, and clonidine) [67]. Loperamide and codeine slow intestinal transit via their actions on opiate receptors. These drugs can be used both in the early and in the maintenance phase after small-bowel resection (4–16 mg of loperamide/d). Metoclopramide, a central and peripheral dopamine type II receptor antagonist, may cause dystonic reactions and extrapyramidal symptoms [68]. Erythromycin, a motilin receptor agonist, is associated with drug interactions, delayed gastric emptying at high doses, and cardiac complications when administered intravenously. Cisapride, a 5-HT3 agonist, is associated with cardiac arrhythmias and sudden death. Despite the potential adverse effects, these medications are commonly and effectively used in pediatric SBS patients. Because small-bowel resections tend to increase the incidence of peptic ulcer disease, H2 receptor blockers and proton pump inhibitors can be used to regulate gastric acid production and reduce the extent of secretory diarrhea. Antacids or sucralfate can also be given by mouth or via a nasogastric tube [69]. Clonidine may help to decrease gastric secretion as well as intestinal motility [70]. After massive bowel resection, digestion of fat is poorly tolerated as a result of bile salt malabsorption, thereby resulting in decreased micelle formation and fat digestion. Gastric hypersecretion can additionally occur after small bowel resection and may reduce nutrient absorption by inactivating pancreatic enzymes. To decrease fat malabsorption, pancreatic enzymes such as Creon® (Solvay, Marietta, Georgia) or Pancrease® (McNeil Pharmaceutical, Spring House, PA) can be initiated. Goals of replacement therapy include reduction of abdominal distension and pain, improved quality and decreased frequency of stool, and objective assessment of weight gain and growth. Standard dosing does not exist although the proposed doses are lower than what it is typically used for the treatment of pancreatic insufficiency [71]. Exogenous supplementation of pancreatic enzymes may facilitate digestion of complex nutrients. For example, pancrelipase improves fat and protein absorption after jejunal resection [72]. Antimicrobials (eg, metronidazole, ciprofloxacin, and rifaximin) can be used to treat bacterial overgrowth and jaundice in cases of prolonged TPN. Probiotics may also be of help to patients with SBS. In general, if diarrhea is not improved symptomatically within 14 days at maximum dosage, improvement is unlikely with further use of probiotics [67]. Patients with minor ileal resections (<100 cm) and watery diarrhea induced by bile salts can be treated with cholestyramine, which will bind the bile salts [73,74]. Bile-salt-binding agents may alleviate cholerheic diarrhea, but will exacerbate steatorrheic diarrhea by binding the already depleted bile acid pool. A trial with cholestyramine may be beneficial in defining if the patient has cholerheic or steatorrheic diarrhea, the former improving and the latter worsening with cholestyramine administration [75]. Because cholestyramine can increase steatorrhea, Sturm et al. state that before using this drug, malabsorption of bile acids should be excluded by measurement of fecal fat or a 75-selenium-labeled taurohomocholic acid test [70]. Long-acting somatostatin and its analogs such as octreotide may increase the absorption of water, sodium, and energy as well as reduce diarrhea by prolonging intestinal transit time. Octreotide can also be useful as an antidiarrheal drug in patients with a high-output jejunostomy or ileostomy and secretory diarrhea; however, there is no significant effect in patients requiring permanent parenteral nutrition. Furthermore, octreotide is expensive. Because of the risk of tachyphylaxis with prolonged use, octreotide may only be useful during the adaptation phase [48]. O'Keefe et al investigated the effect of octreotide in patients with very high-output jejunostomies (about 3 L/day), requiring tremendous amounts of intravenous fluids with parenteral nutritional formula day and night. After 10 days, patients given octreotide 100 μg three times a day subcutaneously had significantly reduced stomal fluid and electrolyte losses. They were less thirsty, needed smaller amounts of oral fluids, gained weight because of better hydration, and had better urine output and renal function. As expected, hormonally stimulated gastric acid and pancreatic lipase secretions were significantly reduced [76].

As previously mentioned, Byrne et al. showed that use of bowel growth–enhancing agents along with an optimal diet can decrease dependence on TPN absorption in individuals with less than 50 cm of jejunum–ileum. They further showed that pharmacologic therapy is predictably able to allow patients with an intestinal length–body weight ratio of approximately 0.5 cm/kg or greater to be free of TPN. In patients dependent on TPN with a ratio of jejunal–ileal length-to-body weight more than 0.5 cm/kg, the need for TPN probably can be eliminated by treatment with growth hormone, glutamine, and a diet containing modified carbohydrate–fat ratios [77]. The strong tendency for patients with SBS to develop metabolic acidosis may be offset by administration of sodium bicarbonate powder, tablets, liquid, or wafers in doses of 8 to 12 g/d for a minimum of 6 months, and as long as 18 to 24 months [78]. Anemia and hypoalbuminemia may be treated with intermittent infusions of human serum albumin and packed erythrocytes.

E. Enhancing Adaptation

An increasing number of factors have been identified that can promote epithelial growth, increase epithelial absorptive function, and affect intestinal growth. Recent clinical trials offer the potential of a new modality to care for such patients. Selection of appropriate patients for these new therapies, and ensuring efficacy of these factors will be important objectives over the next several years [79]. In a pilot study, enteral treatment with epidermal growth factor in pediatric SBS improves nutrient absorption, increases tolerance with enteral feeds and improve the infection rate [80].

Teduglutide (Gattex), an analog of naturally occurring glucagon-like peptide-2 (GLP-2), was approved by the FDA in December 2012 for adults with short-bowel syndrome who are dependent on parenteral support. In the intestine, biologically active GLP-21–33 is secreted from enteroendocrine L-cells of the ileum and colon in response to nutritional, hormonal, and neural stimulation. Human and animal studies have revealed that dietary fiber and short-chain fatty acids, carbohydrates, and fats are potent stimulators of GLP-2 secretion.This agent binds to the GLP-2R receptors located in intestinal subpopulations of enteroendocrine cells, subepithelial myofibroblasts, and enteric neurons of the submucosal and myenteric plexus. Activation of these receptors results in the local release of intestinal mediators that increases intestinal absorptive capacity, resulting in increased fluid and nutrient absorption. GLP-II was administered in a small study [81] involving non-TPN-dependent patients and resulted in slightly increased jejunal villus height, energy, and fluid absorption. Teduglutide was found to be associated with increased villus height and fluid absorption, both of which regressed once the medication was discontinued [82]. FDA approval was based on 2 clinical trials and 2 extension studies of patients randomly assigned to receive teduglutide or placebo. The studies were designed to measure the number of patients who achieved at least 20% reduction in the volume of weekly parenteral nutrition after 20 and 24 weeks of treatment. Patients treated with teduglutide achieved 46% and 63% clinical responses compared with 6% and 30% of patients treated with placebo. [83]. A reduction in the volume of parenteral nutrition (liters per week) after 24 weeks of treatment was also observed. Results showed a mean reduction in parenteral nutrition of 2.5 L/week and 4.4 L/week in teduglutide-treated patients, compared with 0.9 L/week and 2.3 L/week in placebo-treated patients.

Wilmore, Byrne, and colleagues published their results on 87 patients treated with this regimen in *Current Problems in Surgery* in 1997 [84]. After 4 weeks, 52% were completely off parenteral nutrition and an additional 38% had significantly reduced parenteral nutrition requirements. The same group of investigators published results with this regimen, also in 1997, in 45 patients with a jejunoileal remnant less than 50 cm and with a segment of colon remaining in continuity. After 4 weeks on the regimen, 58% were liberated from parenteral nutrition. After a mean follow-up of 1.8 years, this had fallen to 40%. GLP-II was administered in a small study [85] involving non-TPN-dependent patients and resulted in slightly increased jejunal villus height, energy, and fluid absorption. More recently, a synthetic analogue of GLP-II — teduglutide -was found to be associated with increased villus height and fluid absorption, both of which regressed once the medication was discontinued [86].

The benefit associated with this therapy lasted nearly 4 months following completion of the 3 weeks of daily growth-hormone injections. It is also unclear whether "booster" injections will be required. The benefits of this therapy must be weighed against the potential side effects, which include fluid retention and edema, arthralgias, and carpal tunnel syndrome. It is not known whether these therapies would be more effective if administered during the adaptive phase following enterectomy. Initial small studies with growth hormone in patients outside the adaptive period showed marginal, if any [87, 88, 89, 90]. However, a recent double-blind, randomized, controlled trial involving 41 patients with short bowel syndrome showed that the use of growth hormone could reduce TPN by approximately 2 L/week, in addition to the reduction achieved with standard therapy - this translated into a reduction of 1 night of infusion in patients who received growth hormone at 0.1 mg/kg/day for 4 weeks [91]. It is unclear whether these effects were related to improved absorption or to appetite stimulation.

Conclusion

Pediatric short bowel syndrome is a complex and unique problem. A child with SBS has distinctive metabolic needs that must be met by balancing both parenteral and enteral routes to improve the function of the remnant small intestine and and to maintain adequate growth and avoid complications associated with TPN. Given the uniqueness of SBS, special attention is required during each phase of growth and adaptation for each patient. Efforts must be made to deliver a balanced TPN solution, avoid catheter related infections, lower the dose of intravenous lipids, possibly the use omega-3 fatty acids, and advance to enteral nutrition as soon as the patient can tolerate. Additional research is needed to refine the enteral formulas and parenteral macro- and micronutrients for this emerging patient population and to enhance and accelerate intestinal adaptation.

Conflict of Interest

None declared.

References

[1] Ching YA, Gura K, Modi B. Pediatric intestinal failure: nutrition, pharmacologic, and surgical approaches. *ASPEN* 2007;22:653-663.

[2] Vanderhoof JA. Short bowel syndrome. *Neonat Gastroenterol* 1996;23:377-386.

[3] Booth IW, Lander AD. Short bowel syndrome. *Bailliere's Clin Gastroenterol* 1998;12:739-772.

[4] Dudrick SJ, Latifi R. Management of short-bowel syndrome. In: Kirby DF, Dudrick SJ, eds. *Practical handbook of nutrition in clinical practice*. Boca Raton: CRC Press, 1994.

[5] Berger DL, Malt RA. Management of the short gut syndrome. *Adv Surg* 1996; 29:43-57.

[6] Scolapio JS, Fleming CR. Short bowel syndrome. *Gastroenterol Clin North Am*. Jun 1998;27(2):467-479.

[7] Ziegler MM. Short bowel syndrome: remedial features that influence outcome and the duration of parenteral nutrition. *J Pediatr* 1997; 131:335-336.

[8] Scolapio JS. Effect of growth hormone and glutamine on the short bowel: five years later [review]. *Gut* 2000; 47:164-171.

[9] Carbonnel F, Cosnes J, Chevret S, et al. The role of anatomic factors in nutritional autonomy after extensive small bowel resection. *JPEN J Parenter Enteral Nutr*. 1996;20:275-280.

[10] Wilmore DW, Dudrick SJ, Daly JM, et al. The role of nutrition in the adaptation of the small intestine after massive resection. *Surg Gynecol Obstet*. Apr 1971;132:673-680.

[11] 78. Nightingale JM, Lennard-Jones JE, Walker ER, et al. Jejunal efflux in short bowel syndrome. *Lancet*. 1990;336(8718):765-768.

[12] . Scolapio JS, Fleming CR. Short bowel syndrome. *Gastroenterol Clin North Am*. Jun 1998;27:467-479.

[13] Woolf GM, Miller C, Kurian R, et al. Nutritional absorption in short bowel syndrome. Evaluation of fluid, calorie, and divalent cation requirements. *Dig Dis Sci*. 1987;32:8-15.

[14] Matarese LE. Nutrition and fluid optimization for patients with short bowel syndrome. *JPEN J Parenter Enteral Nutr*. 2013;37:161-170.

[15] Williams NS, Evans P, King RFGJ. Gastric acid secretion and gastrin production in the short bowel syndrome. *Gut*. 1985; 26: 914-919.

[16] Buchman AL, Scolapio J, Fryer J. AGA technical review on short bowel syndrome and intestinal transplantation. *Gastroenterology*. 2003; 124: 1111-1134.
[17] da Cunha Ferreira RMC, Cash RA. Treatment and prevention of dehydration in diarrheal disease: a guide for use at the primary level. Geneva, Switzerland: World Health Organization (WHO); 1976.
[18] Lennard-Jones JE. Oral rehydration solutions in short bowel syndrome. *Clin Ther*. 1990; suppA129-137.
[19] Fortran JS, Rector FC Jr, Carter NW. The mechanism of sodium absorption in the human small intestine. *J Clin Invest*. 1968; 47: 884-900.
[20] Davis GR, Santa Ana CA, Morawski SG, Fortran JC. Permeability characteristics of human jejunum, ileum, proximal colon, and distal colon: results of potential difference measurements and unidirectional fluxes. *Gastroenterology*. 1982; 83: 844-850.
[21] Fleming CR, George L, Stoner GL, et al. The importance of urinary magnesium values in patients with gut failure. *Mayo Clin Proc*. 1984; 71: 334-337.
[22] Hylander E, Ladefoged K, Madsen S. Calcium balance and bone mineral content following small-intestinal resection. *Scand J Gastroenterol*. 1981; 16: 167-176.
[23] Nightingale JM, Lennard-Jones JE, Walker ER, Farthing MJ. Oral salt supplements to compensate for jejunostomy losses: comparison of sodium chloride capsules, glucose electrolyte solution, and glucose polymer electrolyte solution. *Gut* 1992; 33:759-761.
[24] Stollman NH, Neustater BR, Rogers AI. Short bowel syndrome. *Gastroenterologist* 1996; 4:118-128.
[25] Andorsky DJ, Lund DP, Lillehei CW, et al. Nutritional and other postoperative management of neonates with short bowel syndrome correlates with clinical outcomes. *J Pediatr* 2001;139:27-33.
[26] Salvino R, Ghanta R, Seidner DL, Mascha E, Xu Y, Steiger E. Liver failure is ncommon in adults receiving long-term parenteral nutrition. *JPEN J Parent Enteral Nutr* 2006; 30:202-208.
[27] Buchman AL. Complications of long-term home total parenteral nutrition: their identification, prevention and treatment. *Dig. Dis. Sci.* 2001;46:1-18.
[28] Collier S, Crouch J, Hendricks K. Use of cyclic parenteral nutrition in infants less than 6 months of age. *Nutr Clin Pract* 1994;9:65-68.

[29] Takehara H, Hino M, Kameoka K. A new method of total parenteral nutrition for surgical neonates: it is possible that cyclic TPN prevents intrahepatic cholestasis. *Tokushima J Exp Med* 1990;37:97-102.

[30] Wretlind A. Development of fat emulsions. *JPEN J Parenter Enteral Nutr* 1981;5:230-235.

[31] Burdge GC, Calder PC. Conversion of alpha-linolenic acid to longer-chain polyunsaturated fatty acids in human adults. *Reprod Nutr Dev* 2005;45:581-597.

[32] Ruxton CHS, Calder PC, Reed SC, Simpson MJA. The impact of long-chain n-3 polyunsaturated fatty acids on human health. *Nutrition Research Reviews*. 2005;18:113-129.

[33] Calder PC. n-3 fatty acids, inflammation, and immunity relevance to postsurgical and critically ill patients. *Lipids* 2004;39:1147-1161.

[34] Le HD, de Meijer VE, Robinson EM, Zurakowski D, Potemkin AK, Arsenault DA, Fallon EM, Malkan A, Bistrian BR, Gura KM, Puder M. Parenteral fish-oil-based lipid emulsion improves fatty acid profiles and lipids in parenteral nutrition-dependent children. *Am J Clin Nutr* 2011; 94:749-758.

[35] Sigalet D, Boctor D, Brindle M, Lam V, Robertson M. Elements of successful intestinal rehabilitation. *J Pediatr Surg* 2011;46:150-156.

[36] Cooper A, Betts JM, Pereira GR. Taurine deficiency in the severe hepatic dysfunction complicating total parenteral nutrition. *J Ped Surg* 1984;19:462-466.

[37] Dahlstrom KA, Ament ME, Laidlaw SA. Plasma amino acid concentrations in children receiving long-term parenteral nutrition. *J Pediatr Gastroenterol Nutr* 1988;7:748-754.

[38] Sondheimer JM, Asturias E, Cadnapaphornchai M. Infection and cholestasis in neonates with intestinal resection and long-term parenteral nutrition. *J Pediatr Gastroenterol Nutr* 1998;27:131-137.

[39] Beath SV, Davies P, Papadopoulou A. Parenteral nutrition-related cholestasis in postsurgical neonates: multivariate analysis of risk factors. *J Pediatr Surg* 1996;31:604-606.

[40] Fratino G, Molinari AC, Mazzola C. Prospective study of indwelling central venous catheter-related complications in children with Broviac or clampless valved catheters. *Hematol Oncol* 2002;24:657-661.

[41] Dannenberg C, Bierbach U, Rothe A. Ethanol-lock technique in the treatment of blood stream infections in pediatric patients oncology patients with Broviac catheter. *J Pediatr Hem Onc* 2003;25:616-21.

[42] Messing B, Peitra-Cohen S, Debure A. Antibiotic-lock technique: a new approach to optimal therapy for catheter related sepsis in home-parenteral nutrition patients. *JPEN* 1988;12:185-189.

[43] Segarra-Newnham M, Martin-Cooper EM. Antibiotic lock technique: a review of the literature. *Ann Pharmacother* 2005;39:311-318.

[44] Al-Hwiesh AK. Tunneled catheter-antibiotic lock therapy for prevention of dialysis catheter-related infections: a single center experience. *Saudi J Kidney Dis Transplant* 2008;19:593-602.

[45] Metcalf SCL, Chambers ST, Pithie AD. Use of ethanol locks to prevent recurrent central line sepsis. *J Infect* 2004;49:20-22.

[46] Broom J, Woods M, Allworth A. Ethanol lock therapy to treat tunneled central venous catheter-associated blood stream infections: results from a prospective trial. *Scand J Infect Dis* 2008;40:399-406.

[47] Mouw E, Chessman K, Lesher A, Tagge E. Use of an ethanol lock to prevent catheter-related infections in children with short bowel syndrome. *J Pediatr Surg* 2008;43:1025-1029.

[48] Scolapio JS. Effect of growth hormone, glutamine, and diet on adaptation in short-bowel syndrome: a randomized, controlled study. *Gastroenterology* 1997; 113:1074-1081.

[49] Skipper A. Dietitian's handbook of enteral and parenteral nutrition. Rockville, MD: Aspen, 1989.

[50] Stump ES. *Nutrition and diagnosis-related care,* 3rd ed. Philadelphia: Lea and Febiger, 1992.

[51] Levy E, Frileux P, Sandrucci S, Ollivier JM, Masini JP, Cosnes J, Hannoun L, Parc R. Continuous enteral nutrition during the early adaptive stage of the short bowel syndrome. *Br J Surg* 1988;75:549-553.

[52] Scolapio JS, Fleming CR. Short-bowel syndrome. *Gastroenterol Clin North Am* 1998; 27:467-479.

[53] Anderson H, Isaksson B, Sjogren B. Fat-reduced diet in the symptomatic treatment of small bowel disease. *Gut* 1997; 15:351-359.

[54] Stringer MD, Puntis JWL. Short bowel syndrome. *Arch. Dis. Child* 1995; 73:170-173.

[55] Nordgaard I, Hansen BS, Mortensen PB. Colon as a digestive organ in patients with short bowel. *Lancet* 1994; 343:373-376.

[56] Koruda MJ, Rolandelli RH, Settle RG, Zimmaro DM, Rombeau JL. Effect of parenteral nutrition supplemented with short-chain fatty acids on adaptation to massive small bowel resection. *Gastroenterology* 1988;95:715-720.

[57] Woolf GM, Miller C, Kurian R, Jeejeebhoy KN. Diet for patients with a short bowel: high fat or high carbohydrate? *Gastroenterology* 1983; 84:823-828.

[58] Woolf GM, Miller C, Kurian R, Jeejeebhoy KN. Nutritional absorption in short bowel syndrome: evaluation of fluid, calories, and divalent cation requirements. *Dig Dis Sci* 1987; 32:8-15.

[59] Sundaram A, Koutkia P, Apovian C. Nutritional Management of Short Bowel Syndrome in Adults. *J Clin Gastroenterol* 2002; 34:207-220.

[60] Hadjittofi C, Coran AG, Mogilner JG, Pollak Y, Matter I, Sukhotnik I. Dietary supplementation with vitamin D stimulates intestinal epithelial cell turnover after massive small bowel resection in rats. *Pediatr Surg Int* 2013;29:41-50.

[61] Fleming R, George L, Stoner GL. The importance of urinary magnesium values in patients with gut failure. *Mayo Clinic Proc.* 1996; 71:21-24.

[62] Klein S, Jeejeebhoy KN. Long-term nutritional management of patients with maldigestion and malabsorption in gastrointestinal disease, 5th ed. Sleisenger M, Fordtran J, eds. Philadelphia: WB Saunders, 1993.

[63] Lennard-Jones JE. Practical management of the short bowel. *Aliment Pharmacol Ther* 1994; 8:563-577.

[64] Ladefoged K, Olgaard K. Sodium homeostasis after small-bowel resection. *Scand J Gastroenterol* 1985; 20:361-369.

[65] Allard JP, Jeejeebhoy KN. Nutritional support and therapy in the short bowel syndrome. *Gastroenterol Clin North Am* 1989; 18:589-601.

[66] Wilmore DW. Growth factors and nutrients in the short bowel syndrome. *JPEN J Parent Enteral Nutr* 1999;23(5 Suppl):S117-120.

[67] Shatnawei A, Parekh NR, Rhoda KM, Speerhas R, Stafford J, Dasari V, Quintini C, Kirby DF, Steiger E. Intestinal failure management at the Cleveland Clinic. *Arch. Surg.* 2010; 145:521-527.

[68] Ching YA, Gura K, Modi B. Pediatric intestinal failure: nutrition, pharmacologic, and surgical approaches. *ASPEN* 2007;22:653-663.

[69] Sturm A, Layer P, Goebell H. Short-bowel syndrome: an update on the therapeutic approach. *Scand. J. Gastroenterol.* 1997; 32:288-296.

[70] Avery MF, Snyder JD. Oral therapy for acute diarrhea: the under-used simple solution. *N. Engl. J. Med.* 1990; 323:891-894.

[71] Stevens T, Conwell D. Pancreatic Enzyme Replacement and Bile Acid Therapy. In: Matarese, LE.; Steiger, E.; Seidner, DL., editors. *Intestinal Failure and Rehabilitation: A Clinical Guide Boca Raton.* CRC Press; 2005. pp 161-172.

[72] Stump ES. *Nutrition and diagnosis-related care*, 3rd ed. Philadelphia: Lea and Febiger, 1992.

[73] Thompson JS. Management of the short bowel syndrome. *Gastroenterol Clin North Am* 1994; 23:403-420.

[74] Berger DL, Malt RA. Management of the short gut syndrome. *Adv Surg* 1996; 29:43-57.

[75] Purdum PP, Kirby DF. Short bowel syndrome: a review of the role of nutrition support. *JPEN J Parenter Enteral Nutr* 1991; 15:93-101.

[76] O'Keefe SJ, Peterson ME, Fleming CR. Octreotide as an adjunct to home parenteral nutrition in the management of permanent end jejunostomy syndrome. *JPEN J Parenter Enteral Nutr* 1994; 18:26-34.

[77] Byrne TA, Persinger RL, Young LS, Ziegler TR, Wilmore DW. New treatment of patients with short bowel syndrome: growth hormone, glutamine, and a modified diet. *Ann Surg* 1995; 222:243-255.

[78] Dudrick SJ, Latifi R. Management of short-bowel syndrome. In: Kirby DF, Dudrick SJ, eds. *Practical handbook of nutrition in clinical practice.* Boca Raton: CRC Press, 1994.

[79] Yang H, Teitelbaum DH. Novel Agents in the Treatment of Intestinal Failure: Humoral Factors. *Gastroenterology* 2006; 130(2 Suppl 1): S117-121.

[80] Sigalet DL, Martin GR, Butzner JD, Buret A, Meddings JB. A pilot study of the use of epidermal growth factor in pediatric short bowel syndrome. *J. Pediatr. Surg.* 2005;40:763-768.

[81] Jeppesen PB, Hartmann B, Thulesen J, et al. Glucagon-like peptide 2 improves nutrient absorption and nutritional status in short-bowel patients with no colon. *Gastroenterology*. 2001; 120: 806-815.

[82] Jeppesen PB, Blosch CM, Lopansri JB, et al. ALX-0600, a dipeptidyl peptidase-IV resistant glucagon-like peptide-2 (GLP-2) analog, improves intestinal function in short bowel syndrome (SBS) patients with a jejunostomy. *Gastroenterology*. 2002; 122: S1249.

[83] Jeppesen PB, Pertkiewicz M, Messing B, Iyer K, Seidner DL, O'keefe SJ, et al. Teduglutide reduces need for parenteral support among patients with short bowel syndrome with intestinal failure. *Gastroenterology*. Dec 2012;143:1473-1481.

[84] Wilmore DW, Byrne TA, Persinger RL. Short bowel syndrome: new therapeutic approaches. *Curr Probl Surg*. May 1997; 34: 389-444.

[85] Jeppesen PB, Hartmann B, Thulesen J, et al. Glucagon-like peptide 2 improves nutrient absorption and nutritional status in short-bowel patients with no colon. *Gastroenterology*. 2001; 120: 806-815.

[86] Jeppesen PB, Blosch CM, Lopansri JB, et al. ALX-0600, a dipeptidyl peptidase-IV resistant glucagon-like peptide-2 (GLP-2) analog, improves intestinal function in short bowel syndrome (SBS) patients with a jejunostomy. *Gastroenterology*. 2002; 122: S1249.

[87] Szkudlarek J, Jeppesen PB, Mortensen PB. Effect of high dose growth hormone with glutamine and no change in diet on intestinal absorption in short bowel patients: a randomized, double-blind, crossover, placebo-controlled study. *Gut*. 2000; 47: 199-205.

[88] Scolapio JS, Camilleri M, Fleming CR, et al. Effect of growth hormone, glutamine, and diet on adaptation in short bowel syndrome: a randomized, controlled trial. *Gastroenterology*. 1997; 113: 1074-1081.

[89] Ellegard L, Bosaeus I, Nordgren S, Bengtsson BA. Low-dose recombinant human growth hormone increases body weight and lean body mass in patients with short bowel syndrome. *Ann Surg*. 1997; 225: 88-96.

[90] Seguy D, Vahedi K, Kapel N, et al. Low dose growth hormone in adult home parenteral nutrition-dependent short bowel syndrome patients: a positive study. *Gastroenterology*. 2003; 124: 293-302.

[91] Byrne TA, Lautz DB, Iyer KR, et al. Recombinant human growth hormone (rhGH) reduces parenteral nutrition in patients with short bowel syndrome: a prospective, randomized, double-blind, placebo-controlled trial. *J Parenter Enteral Nutr*. 2003; 27: S17.

In: Short Bowel Syndrome in Children
Editor: Igor Sukhotnik
ISBN: 978-1-62948-518-8

Chapter VII

Novel Agents in the Treatment of Intestinal Failure: Humoral Factors

Bhani Chawla, M.D., Yongjia Feng, M.D., Ph.D. and Daniel H. Teitelbaum, M.D.*

C.S. Mott Children's Hospital,
University of Michigan Hospital and Health Systems, Ann Arbor, MI, US

Abstract

The goal of medical management of short bowel syndrome is to optimize intestinal adaptation with the hope of weaning off of or avoiding parenteral nutrition dependence. While the patient suffering from a loss of intestine will undergo a series of adaptive responses, including increases in intestinal mass, diameter and length, this may be insufficient to allow for the patient to full wean from parenteral nutrition (PN). Multiple hormones have been noted to stimulate intestinal growth. The three best studied, human growth hormone, epidermal growth factor and GLP-2, are detailed herein.

* Corresponding author: Daniel H. Teitelbaum, M.D., Section of Pediatric Surgery, University of Michigan, CS Mott Children's Hospital 1540 E. Hospital Dr., SPC 4211, Ann Arbor, MI 48109-4211 Phone: +1-734-936-8464. Fax: +1-734-936-9784. E-mail: dttlbm@umich.edu.

Introduction

The management of children with short bowel syndrome (SBS) presents numerous challenges for physicians and other health care professionals. Management goals should include appropriate and timely initiation of parenteral and enteral nutrition as well as different hormones and peptide growth factors that promote optimal intestinal adaptation and continue growth and development. Multiple hormones have been noted to stimulate intestinal adaptation. The three best studied, human growth hormone, epidermal growth factor and GLP-2, are detailed herein.

I. Growth Hormone

Growth hormone (GH) is produced in the anterior pituitary gland, and acts by binding to GH receptors on target cells in multiple systems to promote growth and anabolism. GH is best known for stimulating bone growth, but also stimulates muscle growth, lipolysis, protein synthesis, gluconeogenesis, and helps maintain overall homeostasis [1,2]. GH is regulated by multiple factors including a negative feedback mechanism by circulating levels of IGF-1, the main effector of Growth hormone [3].

a. Animal Studies

As early as the 1950s, hypophysectomy was recognized to have negative effects on the gastrointestinal tract including decreased mitosis, mucosal atrophy, decreased cell mass, and impaired absorptive ability [4]. Multiple studies have shown in rodents after bowel resection, use of GH, with and without glutamine, improves small bowel growth [1,5-7]. Structurally, by increasing cellular proliferation and functionally by increasing absorption of water, electrolytes, and nutrients [8]. The effects of GH on intestinal adaptation are thought to be mediated primarily by the local effects of IGF-1. Exogenous GH administration increases both serum and local intestinal IGF-1 levels [5,6]. Within the jejunum in a rat modelonly IGF-1, not GH, stimulates mucosal growth [9] and is able to reverse the effects of TPN induced mucosal atrophy [10].

There are some studies, however, that argue adding GH does not affect mucosal growth after resection. Rather, the changes seen are only normal adaptive responses to bowel resection [11,12]. Bowel from GH-deficient rats exhibit the same level of mucosal hyperplasia as wild-type.[12] Overall, animal studies appeared to show a functional benefit to use of GH with and with-out glutamine, leading to interest in human studies and eventually FDA approval for use in Short Bowel Syndrome (SBS) in 2003 [13].

b. Clinical Studies in Favor of

Similar to animal studies, clinical trials have also been controversial. Byrne et al., in 1995 including 47 patients, was one of the first studies to look at GH in SBS adults. In this open crossover study, patients were placed on a regimen including a GH, astructured high-carbohydrate, low fat diet and the amino acid glutamine. This regimen resulted in increased nutrient absorption and decreased stool output. After 4 weeks, 57% of the treated patients were weaned off of parenteral nutrition, and 40% of the treated patients remained off of PN at one year. Side effects noted were mainly peripheral edema and arthralgias [14]. Another open-label study by the same group evaluated 61 patients treated with a variable dose of GH (mean 0.09mg/kg/day) along with glutamine and diet that varied based on the presence or absence of a colon. Treatment lasted 4-6 weeks, and 41% percent of the PN dependent patients at the onset of the study remained PN-free at 1 year [15]. One critique of these studies is that there may have been duplication between these two studies [16].

Byrne et al., continued on to publish a double blinded, placebo controlled randomized trial in 2005 [17]. There were three treatment arms: oral glutamine + HGH placebo, oral glutamine placebo + HGH, and both oral glutamine + HGH. Forty one patients were involved and treated over a 4 week period. The primary outcome was reduction in PN requirements. After 3 months of follow-up, only patients that received both glutamine and HGH had statistically significant decrease in PN use. Peripheral edema was again noted to be the most significant side effect.

Seguy et al. 2003 performed a cross-over study in 12 patients who were randomized to receive GH or placebo over 3 weeks with one week wash-out period prior to crossing over to the other treatment arm. Findings included increased weight gain and lean body mass during the treatment period, along with increased absorption of energy, carbohydrates, and nitrogen [18].

Open-label trials have also been conducted in the pediatric population. One small study, Guo et al., 2012 reported favorably weaning off of PN by 6/7 of the participants given a regimen including GH, glutamine, and a high-carbohydrate, low fat diet. The effects were sustained after cessation of treatment with GH as well [19].

a. *Clinical Studies Equivocal or Against*

Ellegard et al., 1997 conducteda randomized, double-blind, placebo-controlled crossover study that can best be categorized as equivocal. Tenparticipants were randomized to receive either GH or a placebo. Only twopatients were PN dependent at the start of the study. While on treatment with GH for 8 weeks, patients demonstrated weight gain and increased lean body mass. These effects disappeared, however, over the next few months during the wash-out period (12 weeks) [20]. Two other randomized control trials also did not have exhibit favorable outcomes. Scolapio et al., 1997 also performed a randomized, double-blind, placebo controlled crossover study involving 8 patients. Patients received GH and glutamine or placebo for 21 days before switching to the other arm of treatment, in addition to receiving a high-carbohydrate, low fat diet. In this study, patients were noted to have transiently increased weight and lean body mass similar to that reported by both Ellegard et al., and Seguy et al. However, the authors of this study concluded negatively about the use of GH treatment as no sustained weight gain and no changes in nutrient absorption were observed [21]. Szkudlarek et al., 2000 performed a similarly designed cross-over study with 8 patients randomized to receive GH and glutamine or placebo for 4 weeks. There was, however, no change in diet. The outcome measures of this study were macronutrient absorption. There were no significant changes [22]. A pediatric study, Peretti et al., 2011 studied 14 PN dependent patients randomized to two arms: 4 months of GH or 4 months with-out treatment followed by cross-over to 4 months of GH. During the trial period, PN was being actively weaned. There was no sustained benefit noted from use of GH [23]. In conclusion, while HGH is approved by the FDA for SBS patients, it is difficult to advocate for the use of this growth factor at this time.

II. Epidermal Growth Factor

Epidermal growth factor (EGF) is one of the most potent factors for driving epithelial cell growth with the GI tract. Animal data strongly supports the use of EGF family of factors. EGF treated SBS rats had reduced weight loss, improved carbohydrate absorption and reduced intestinal permeability [24]. Use of another EGF-family member, transforming growth factor-alpha (TGF-α), has also shown significant improvement in intestinal adaptation in a rat SBS model [25].

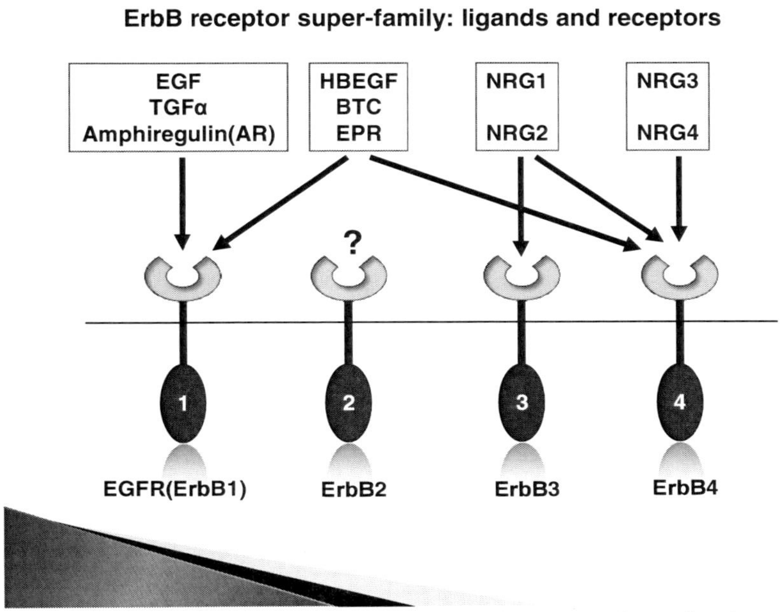

The first group of ligands includes EGF, amphiregulin (AR), and transforming growth factor-α (TGF-α), which bind specifically to EGFR; the second group includes betacellulin (BTC), heparin-binding EGF (HB-EGF), and epiregulin(EPR), which exhibit dual specificity in that they bind both EGFR and ErbB4.

Figure 1. Growth factors signal through one or more of 4 ErbB receptor super family members on the EC surface, and typically will co-dimerize with two different receptors to effect its action.

Despite the strong animal data, relatively few clinical studies have been performed. The most concrete evidence that EGF may have benefit on a clinical level was a pilot study performed by Sigalet, et al., [26]. In this trial, five patients with severe SBS (all less than 25% of their predicted length for gestational age were prospectively treated with 100 μg/kg/day of human recombinant EGF. Interestingly, all showed significant improvement in carbohydrate absorption and improved enteral feeding tolerance. While no adverse events occurred during the administration phase, 3 out of the 5 patients become septic within 2 weeks of EGF discontinuation. Clearly, the study has some promising results, but larger trials and a wider examination of safety issues will be needed.

III. Experimental Growth Factors

Several growth factors have been hypothesized to drive intestinal growth, but have not been trialed in humans. Two potential factors include the use of heparin-bound EGF [27] as well as orally administered insulin [28]. While the mechanisms of these factors may seem distinct, these two factors, as well as transforming growth factor – alpha all drive growth signals through EGF-like signaling pathways [29]. Clearly, determining which of these may have the most impact in a clinical setting remains to be determined. Growth factors signal through one or more of 4 ErbB receptor super family members on the epithelial cell surface, and typically will co-dimerize with two different receptors to effect its action (Figure 1).

The first group of ligands includes EGF, amphiregulin (AR), and transforming growth factor-α (TGF-α), which bind specifically to EGFR; the second group includes betacellulin (BTC), heparin-binding EGF (HB-EGF), and epiregulin(EPR), which exhibit dual specificity in that they bind both EGFR and ErbB4.

IV. Glucagon Like Peptide-2/Teduglutide

Glucagon-like peptide-2 is produced endogenously in L cells of the ileum and colon [30]. Functions include facilitating growth of normal intestinal epithelium, increasing intestinal blood flow, slowing gastric emptying, and reducing gastric secretions; in addition it is noted to have anti-inflammatory properties [31]. These actions which so closely target the consequences of short bowel syndrome, led to interest in GLP-2 as a treatment option. [3] Studies in both animals and humans have been promising. Teduglutide, a GLP-2 analog, is newly approved by the FDA for the treatment of short bowel syndrome since December of 2012 [32].

a. Animal Studies

Studies in rodent and pig models have shown GLP-2 to have a significant effect on adaptive changes that occur after resection [33-39]. Rats that have undergone massive bowel resection have higher plasma levels of GLP-2 [35-36]. In addition, in a porcine model of parenteral nutrition, GLP-2 increased intestinal blood flow [40]. In unresected mice, exogenous administration of GLP-2 leads to increases in small bowel mass, crypt cell proliferation, mucosal thickness, and reduced apoptosis [33,34]. Administration of GLP-2 produces similar changes, amplifying trophic adaption in both rodents and pigs after massive bowel resection [37-39,41]. Some of this effect may be explained by amplification of endogenous GLP-2 action. Exogenous human GLP-2 given to rats after major resection was found to actually increase the expression of GLP-2 receptor by 3-fold in the ileum [42]. Interestingly, like GH GLP-2's enterotrophic effects may also be mediated by IGF-1 [43.44].

b. Clinical Studies in Favor of GLP-2 Derivatives

One of the earliest positive studies in human subjects was conducted by Jeppensen et al., in 2001 [45]. Eight short gut patients, four of whom were TPN dependent, received GLP-2 for 35days. Based on measurements before and after, patients gained weight and lean body mass, had delayed gasric emptying and increased energy absorption. Microscopically, increases of crypt depth and villus height were also demonstrated. Another physiologic change induced by GLP-2 administration in an increase in post-prandial mesenteric blood flow. This has been demonstrated in both healthy volunteers and short gut patients [46,47].

Teduglutide became of interest as a substitute for GLP-2 because of its prolonged half-life. GLP-2's half-life is only seven minutes due to rapid digestion by the enzyme dipeptidyl peptidase IV(DPPIV). Teduglutide is resistant to DPPIV by differing from GLP-2 by only one amino acid. This change extends the half-life to over 2 hours [3]. An open-label phase II study also by Jeppensen et al., in 2005 in 16 short gut patients showed similar findings of increased wet weight and energy absorption [48].

The same group continued on to establish the clinical efficacy of teduglutide in two larger double-blind, placebo-controlled, multicenter, randomized phase III clinical trials [49,50]. It was interesting that the first phase III trial demonstrated more benefit with the lower dosing of Teduglutide (0.05 mg/kg/d), and thus the second phase III trial used this lower dose. Results from this latter 24-week trial of adult SBS patients showed that Teduglutide was superior to placebo in several outcomes. In particular, volume of parenteral nutrition solution was significantly reduced. In fact, this reduction came quickly in the treated group, where a mean of 4.4 liters per week were reduced (2-fold better than placebo). Approximately 54% of patients had a reduction in days of TPN, and a significant increase in plasma citrulline, a biomarker of functional intestinal epithelial cell mass, was noted in the Teduglutide group.

Long-term outcomes are just coming out. At 52 weeks of treatment, only 7 patients, out of 52 withdrew due to adverse events, mostly due to GI disorders

[51], and mostly in those with more than 100 cm of intestine. In general, the safety record in these patients was strikingly good.

An interesting follow up study was recently reported where the patient's quality of life (QOL) scores were compared in those study patients [52]. Those patients experiencing reductions in their PN experienced an improvement in these QOL scores. The changes, however, were not statistically different from the placebo group, and thus, more studies on larger numbers of patients may be needed to more fully understand the true impact of Teduglutide on this important factor.

In conclusion, the use of several new growth factors, particularly GLP-2, may have striking benefits to SBS patients. It will be exciting to see if these positive effects will be similarly found once such clinical trials will be applied to the pediatric population with SBS. A strong word of caution needs to be given with the use of any of these growth factors. For many patients the use of these will be costly and often needed long-term. More importantly, animal studies have suggested that GLP-2 can promote pre-neoplastic polyps [53]. The safety of using these agents has not been tested beyond 52 weeks. It will be important to follow these patients longer to make sure that they do not develop the formation of polyps or neoplastic conditions.

References

[1] Zhou, X; Li, YX; Li, N; Li, JS. Glutamine enhances the gut-trophic effect of growth hormone in rat after massive small bowel resection. *J Surg Res.*, Jul 2001, 99(1), 47-52.

[2] Krysiak, R; Gdula-Dymek, A; Bednarska-Czerwinska, A; Okopien B. Growth hormone therapy in children and adults. *Pharmacol Rep.*, Sep-Oct 2007, 59(5), 500-516.

[3] Pereira, PM; Bines, JE. New growth factor therapies aimed at improving intestinal adaptation in short bowel syndrome. *J Gastroenterol Hepatol.*, Jun 2006, 21(6), 932-940.

[4] Schapiro, H; Wruble, LD; Britt, LG. The effect of hypophysectomy on the gastrointestinal tract. A review of the literature. *Am J Dig Dis.*, Nov 1970, 15(11), 1019-1030.

[5] Lund, PK. Molecular basis of intestinal adaptation: the role of the insulin-like growth factor system. *Ann N Y Acad Sci.*, Nov 17 1998, 859, 18-36.

[6] Lund, PK; Ulshen, MH; Rountree, DB; Selub, SE; Buchan, AM. Molecular biology of gastrointestinal peptides and growth factors: relevance to intestinal adaptation. *Digestion.*, 1990, 46, Suppl 2:66-73.

[7] Gu, Y; Wu, ZH; Xie, JX; Jin, DY; Zhuo, HC. Effects of growth hormone (rhGH) and glutamine supplemented parenteral nutrition on intestinal adaptation in short bowel rats. *Clin Nutr.*, Apr 2001, 20(2), 159-166.

[8] Cisler, JJ; Buchman, AL. Intestinal adaptation in short bowel syndrome. *J Investig Med.*, Dec 2005, 53(8), 402-413.

[9] Lo, HC; Ney, DM GH; and IGF-I differentially increase protein synthesis in skeletal muscle and jejunum of parenterally fed rats. *Am J Physiol.*, Nov 1996, 271(5 Pt 1), E872-878.

[10] Peterson, CA; Carey, HV; Hinton, PL; Lo, HC; Ney, DM. GH elevates serum IGF-I levels but does not alter mucosal atrophy in parenterally fed rats. *Am J Physiol.*, May 1997, 272(5 Pt 1), G1100-1108.

[11] Park, JH; Vanderhoof, JA. Growth hormone did not enhance mucosal hyperplasia after small-bowel resection. *Scand J Gastroenterol.*, Apr 1996, 31(4), 349-354.

[12] Durant, M; Gargosky, S; Dahlstrom, K; Fang, R; Hellman, B; Jr. Castillo, R. The role of growth hormone in adaptation to massive small intestinal resection in rats. *Pediatr Res.*, Feb 2001, 49(2), 189-196.

[13] Franklin, SL; Geffner, ME. Growth hormone: the expansion of available products and indications. *Endocrinol Metab Clin North Am.*, Sep 2009, 38(3), 587-611.

[14] Byrne, TA; Persinger, RL; Young, LS; Ziegler, TR; Wilmore, DW. A new treatment for patients with short-bowel syndrome. Growth hormone, glutamine, and a modified diet. *Ann Surg.*, Sep 1995, 222(3), 243-254, discussion 254-245.

[15] Byrne, TA; Cox, S; Karimbakas, M; et al. Bowel rehabilitation: an alternative to long-term parenteral nutrition and intestinal transplantation for some patients with short bowel syndrome. *Transplant Proc.*, May 2002, 34(3), 887-890.

[16] Messing, B; Blethen, S; Dibaise, JK; Matarese, LE; Steiger, E. Treatment of adult short bowel syndrome with recombinant human growth hormone: a review of clinical studies. *J Clin Gastroenterol.*, May-Jun 2006, 40 Suppl 2, S75-84.

[17] Byrne, TA; Wilmore, DW; Iyer, K; et al. Growth hormone, glutamine, and an optimal diet reduces parenteral nutrition in patients with short

bowel syndrome: a prospective, randomized, placebo-controlled, double-blind clinical trial. *Ann Surg.*, Nov 2005, 242(5), 655-661.

[18] Seguy, D; Vahedi, K; Kapel, N; Souberbielle, JC; Messing, B. Low-dose growth hormone in adult home parenteral nutrition-dependent short bowel syndrome patients: a positive study. *Gastroenterology.*, Feb 2003, 124(2), 293-302.

[19] Guo; M; Li, Y; Li, J. Role of growth hormone, glutamine and enteral nutrition in pediatric short bowel syndrome: a pilot follow-up study. *Eur J Pediatr Surg.*, Apr 2012, 22(2), 121-126.

[20] Ellegard, L; Bosaeus, I; Nordgren, S; Bengtsson, BA. Low-dose recombinant human growth hormone increases body weight and lean body mass in patients with short bowel syndrome. *Ann Surg.*, Jan 1997, 225(1), 88-96.

[21] Scolapio, JS; Camilleri, M; Fleming, CR; et al. Effect of growth hormone, glutamine, and diet on adaptation in short-bowel syndrome: a randomized, controlled study. *Gastroenterology.*, Oct 1997,113(4), 1074-1081.

[22] Szkudlarek; J; Jeppesen, PB; Mortensen, PB. Effect of high dose growth hormone with glutamine and no change in diet on intestinal absorption in short bowel patients: a randomised, double blind, crossover, placebo controlled study. *Gut.*, Aug 2000, 47(2), 199-205.

[23] Peretti, N; Loras-Duclaux, I; Kassai, B; et al. Growth hormone to improve short bowel syndrome intestinal autonomy: a pediatric randomized open-label clinical trial. *JPEN J Parenter Enteral Nutr.*, Nov 2011, 35(6), 723-731.

[24] Sham, J; Martin, G; Meddings, JB; Sigalet, DL. Epidermal growth factor improves nutritional outcome in a rat model of short bowel syndrome. *J Pediatr Surg.*, May 2002, 37(5), 765-769.

[25] Sukhotnik, I; Yakirevich, E; Coran, AG; et al. Effect of transforming growth factor-alpha on intestinal adaptation in a rat model of short bowel syndrome. *J Surg Res.*, Dec 2002, 108(2), 235-242.

[26] Sigalet, DL; Martin, GR; Butzner, JD; Buret, A; Meddings, JB. A pilot study of the use of epidermal growth factor in pediatric short bowel syndrome. *J Pediatr Surg.*, May 2005, 40(5), 763-768.

[27] Xia, G; Martin, AE; Michalsky, MP; Besner, GE. Heparin-binding EGF-like growth factor preserves crypt cell proliferation and decreases bacterial translocation after intestinal ischemia/reperfusion injury. *J Pediatr Surg.*, Jul 2002, 37(7), 1081-1087, discussion 1081-1087.

[28] Ben Lulu, S; Coran, AG; Shehadeh, N; Shamir, R; Mogilner, JG; Sukhotnik, I. Oral insulin stimulates intestinal epithelial cell turnover following massive small bowel resection in a rat and a cell culture model. *Pediatr Surg Int.*, Feb 2012, 28(2), 179-187.

[29] Sukhotnik, I; Shteinberg, D; Ben Lulu, S; et al. Effect of transforming growth factor-alpha on enterocyte apoptosis is correlated with EGF receptor expression along the villus-crypt axis during methotrexate-induced intestinal mucositis in a rat. *Apoptosis.*, 2008, 13(11), 1344-1355.

[30] Estall, JL; Drucker, DJ. Glucagon-like Peptide-2. *Annu Rev Nutr.*, 2006, 26, 391-411.

[31] Dube, PE; Brubaker, PL. Frontiers in glucagon-like peptide-2: multiple actions, multiple mediators. *Am J Physiol Endocrinol Metab.*, Aug 2007, 293(2), E460-465.

[32] Seidner, DL; Schwartz, LK; Winkler, MF; Jeejeebhoy, K; Boullata, JI; Tappenden, KA. Increased intestinal absorption in the era of teduglutide and its impact on management strategies in patients with short bowel syndrome-associated intestinal failure. *JPEN J Parenter Enteral Nutr.*, Mar 2013, 37(2), 201-211.

[33] Drucker, DJ; Erlich, P; Asa, SL; Brubaker, PL. Induction of intestinal epithelial proliferation by glucagon-like peptide 2. *Proc Natl Acad Sci U S A.*, Jul 23 1996, 93(15), 7911-7916.

[34] Tsai, CH; Hill, M; Asa, SL; Brubaker, PL; Drucker, DJ. Intestinal growth-promoting properties of glucagon-like peptide-2 in mice. *Am J Physiol.*, Jul 1997, 273(1 Pt 1), E77-84.

[35] Muto, M; Kaji, T; Mukai, M; et al. Ghrelin and glucagon-like peptide-2 increase immediately following massive small bowel resection. *Peptides.*, May 2013, 43, 160-166.

[36] Ljungmann, K; Hartmann, B; Kissmeyer-Nielsen, P; Flyvbjerg, A; Holst, JJ; Laurberg, S. Time-dependent intestinal adaptation and GLP-2 alterations after small bowel resection in rats. *Am J Physiol Gastrointest Liver Physiol.*, Sep 2001, 281(3), G779-785.

[37] Martin, GR; Wallace, LE; Hartmann, B; et al. Nutrient-stimulated GLP-2 release and crypt cell proliferation in experimental short bowel syndrome. *Am J Physiol Gastrointest Liver Physiol.*, Mar 2005, 288(3), G431-438.

[38] Martin, GR; Wallace, LE; Sigalet, DL. Glucagon-like peptide-2 induces intestinal adaptation in parenterally fed rats with short bowel syndrome. *Am J Physiol Gastrointest Liver Physiol.*, Jun 2004, 286(6), G964-972.

[39] Vegge, A; Thymann, T; Lund, P; et al. Glucagon-Like Peptide-2 Induces Rapid Digestive Adaptation Following Intestinal Resection in Preterm Neonates. *Am J Physiol Gastrointest Liver Physiol.*, Jun 13 2013.

[40] Guan, X; Stoll, B; Lu, X; et al. GLP-2-mediated up-regulation of intestinal blood flow and glucose uptake is nitric oxide-dependent in TPN-fed piglets 1. *Gastroenterology.*, Jul 2003,125(1), 136-147.

[41] Scott, RB; Kirk, D; MacNaughton ,WK; Meddings, JB. GLP-2 augments the adaptive response to massive intestinal resection in rat. *Am J Physiol.*, Nov 1998, 275(5 Pt 1), G911-921.

[42] Koopmann, MC; Nelson, DW; Murali, SG; et al. Exogenous glucagon-like peptide-2 (GLP-2) augments GLP-2 receptor mRNA and maintains proglucagon mRNA levels in resected rats. *JPEN J Parenter Enteral Nutr.*, May-Jun 2008, 32(3), 254-265.

[43] Dube, PE; Rowland, KJ; Brubaker, PL. Glucagon-like peptide-2 activates beta-catenin signaling in the mouse intestinal crypt: role of insulin-like growth factor-I. *Endocrinology.*, Jan 2008, 149(1), 291-301.

[44] Bortvedt, SF; Lund, PK. Insulin-like growth factor 1: common mediator of multiple enterotrophic hormones and growth factors. *Curr Opin Gastroenterol.*, Mar 2012, 28(2), 89-98.

[45] Jeppesen, PB; Hartmann, B; Thulesen, J; et al. Glucagon-like peptide 2 improves nutrient absorption and nutritional status in short-bowel patients with no colon. *Gastroenterology.*, Mar 2001, 120(4), 806-815.

[46] Bremholm, L; Hornum, M; Henriksen, BM; Larsen, S; Holst, JJ. Glucagon-like peptide-2 increases mesenteric blood flow in humans. *Scand J Gastroenterol.*, 2009, 44(3), 314-319.

[47] Bremholm; L, Hornum, M; Andersen, UB; Hartmann, B; Holst, JJ; Jeppesen, PB. The effect of Glucagon-Like Peptide-2 on mesenteric blood flow and cardiac parameters in end-jejunostomy short bowel patients. *Regul Pept.*, Jun 7 2011, 168(1-3), 32-38.

[48] Jeppesen, PB; Sanguinetti, EL; Buchman, A; et al. Teduglutide (ALX-0600), a dipeptidyl peptidase IV resistant glucagon-like peptide 2 analogue, improves intestinal function in short bowel syndrome patients. *Gut.*, Sep 2005, 54(9), 1224-1231.

[49] Jeppesen, PB; Gilroy, R; Pertkiewicz, M; Allard, JP; Messing, B; O'Keefe, SJ. Randomised placebo-controlled trial of teduglutide in reducing parenteral nutrition and/or intravenous fluid requirements in patients with short bowel syndrome. *Gut.*, Jul 2011, 60(7), 902-914.

[50] Jeppesen, PB; Pertkiewicz, M; Messing, B; et al. Teduglutide reduces need for parenteral support among patients with short bowel syndrome

with intestinal failure. *Gastroenterology.*, Dec 2012, 143(6), 1473-1481 e1473.

[51] O'Keefe, SJ; Jeppesen, PB; Gilroy, R; Pertkiewicz, M; Allard, JP; Messing, B. Safety and efficacy of teduglutide after 52 weeks of treatment in patients with short bowel intestinal failure. *Clin Gastroenterol Hepatol.*, Jul 2013, 11(7), 815-823 e813.

[52] Jeppesen, PB; Pertkiewicz, M; Forbes, A; et al. Quality of life in patients with short bowel syndrome treated with the new glucagon-like peptide-2 analogue teduglutide - Analyses from a randomised, placebo-controlled study. *Clin Nutr.*, Mar 28, 2013.

[53] Trivedi, S; Wiber, SC; El-Zimaity, HM; Brubaker, PL. Glucagon-like peptide-2 increases dysplasia in rodent models of colon cancer. *Am J Physiol Gastrointest Liver Physiol.*, Apr 15 2012, 302(8), G840-849.

In: Short Bowel Syndrome in Children
Editor: Igor Sukhotnik ISBN: 978-1-62948-518-8

Chapter VIII

The World Experience of the Pediatric Intestinal Failure Program: Successful Outcomes from Intestinal Rehabilitation

***Amnon Rofe, M.D.*[1] *and I. Sukhotnik, M.D.*[2*]**
[1]Department of Medical Management
[2]Department of Pediatric Surgery
Bnai Zion Medical Center, Technion-Israel Institute of Technology,
The Ruth and Bruce Rappaport Faculty of Medicine, Haifa, Israel

Abstract

Short bowel syndrome is a condition whose treatment requires advanced knowledge and techniques and a multidisciplinary approach. SBS is the endpoint of many intestinal diseases and may result in full recovery, in life-long parenteral nutrition, or in the death of the child. Management of children with SBS is optimized by interdisciplinary coordination of parenteral and enteral nutrition support, medical management of associated complications, surgical lengthening

* Corresponding author: Igor Sukhotnik, MD, Dept Pediatric Surgery B, Bnai Zion Medical Center, 47 Golomb St., P.O.B. 4940, Haifa, 31048, Israel, Ph (h): 972-4-8256815, Ph (b): 972-4-8359647, Fax-972-4-8359620. E-mail: igor-dr@internet-zahav.net.

procedures, and intestinal transplantation. Pediatric Intestinal Failure Centers were established in 14 pediatric hospitals throughout the United States and Canada and Pediatric Intestinal Failure Consortium has been developed and is implementing prospective, multi-institutional studies to better define the specific aspects of intestinal failure management that optimize long-term out comes. The published data from these studies suggest that intestinal failure in pediatric patients is quite treatable and provide further evidence that all infants at risk for intestinal failure should be treated aggressively and referred early to a dedicated intestinal rehabilitation center. Improved communication and integration with the transplant service have resulted in earlier assessment, increased rates of transplantation, and decreased mortality from liver failure. The presented data demonstrate that a newly established intestinal failure program can achieve excellent survival in a cohort of chronically ill and complicated children that has historically been associated with substantial mortality.

Keywords: Short bowel syndrome, intestinal failure, intestinal rehabilitation, program

Introduction

Short bowel syndrome (SBS) is defined as an intestinal failure following the loss of intestinal length or competence below the minimal amount necessary for the digestion and absorption of nutrients that are needed to promote appropriate growth of the infant and to maintain normal nutritional status in adult [1-7]. Despite the evolution of liver and intestinal transplantation, the availability of total parenteral nutrition (TPN), advances in resuscitation, availability of potent antibiotics, and modern techniques of organ support, the morbidity of SBS remains strikingly high [8]. Risk factors that contribute to the high mortality and morbidity include the length of remaining intestine, loss of ileocecal valve, failure to thrive, catheter-related sepsis, and total parenteral nutrition (TPN)-associated cholestasis [9]. Bacterial complications and end-stage liver failure seem to be the most serious complications of SBS, representing the final cause of death in a majority of fatal cases [10]. However, rare complications also have been described. They include D-lactic acidosis, renal and gallbladder stones, gut colitis etc. Until 30 years ago, the prognosis after extensive bowel resection was poor, especially in the neonatal period [11]. The onset of parenteral and enteral feeding in the daily practice has transformed the outcome during the past decades [12]. More than 90% of infants and children now survive after extensive small bowel resection in the neonatal period.

An appropriate management of SBS requires reference centers using therapeutic strategies based on a multidisciplinary approach including pediatric gastroenterologists and pediatric surgeons, as well as specialized nurses, dieticians, social workers, and psychologists. This integrated approach should be adapted to each type and stage of intestinal failure including the home PN and transplantation program. Intestinal rehabilitation to enhance intestinal absorption and function through diet and medication is another therapy that can be used in hopes of weaning parenteral nutrition and preventing malnutrition. Few centers manage all the stages of intestinal failure from onset to intestinal transplantation, including the home PN program. A marked discrepancy has been reported in clinical status between children referred for intestinal transplantation from centers with and without nutritional care teams. Long-term management of intestinal failure has become a very important concern as suggested by recently published articles. A national or international network might provide data on IF on which the needs for health care should be based. In addition, such a network should allow us to optimize the management, to upgrade the medical approach, and to promote basic and applied research in the field [13].

Historically, it was not until the 1990s that serious consideration was given to a coordinated approach to intestinal failure using a team of medical and surgical caregivers [14]. The benefits of a multi-disciplinary approach include the integration of expert management to improve the outcome of the disease process, amalgamation of expert care, a holistic approach to patients, stream-lined diagnosis and treatment, strengthened communication with both, families and the care teams, consistent follow up and continuity of patient care throughout all treatment options.. Several pediatric institutions across North America and Europe have developed comprehensive, multi-disciplinary teams for the treatment and rehabilitation of children with intestinal failure. Goulet and Ruemmele [15] concurred that such teams must be capable of being involved in all aspects of the management of children with intestinal failure. The success of these teams depends on a high level of expertise in pediatric gastroenterology and clinical nutrition, a well-organized home parenteral nutrition (HPN) program, and pediatric surgeons capable of performing both nontransplant pediatric surgery and intestinal transplantation. These will allow, according to Fishbein et al., [16], for optimal individualized care to be given across the spectrum from intestinal rehabilitation when feasible, to transplantation when nutritional recovery is not believed to be achievable. The survival of tens of thousands of children and adults with complicated gastrointestinal problems has been possible because of the pioneering work started by Dudrick as a surgical resident at the Hospital of the University of Pennsylvania [17]. His determination, hard work, and ingenuity have given a valuable tool to help the patients through critical gastrointestinal crises. Treatment strategies have now evolved so that several institutions, especially on the pediatric level, are developing formal, multidisciplinary programs that specialize in the treatment of patients with intestinal failure. Indeed, recent data show that a multidisciplinary approach to intestinal failure may be associated with a reduced rate of mortality. The objective of this chapter was to review the evidence for the benefit of multi-disciplinary teams in the management and outcomes of pediatric patients with intestinal failure.

The World Experience of Pediatric Intestinal Failure Program (IRP)

The Intestinal Care Clinic (ICC) at the Children's Hospital of Pittsburgh was established in December 1996, and serves as a regional, national, and international referral center for patients with SBS [18]. The ICC center is staffed by an interdisciplinary team of pediatric specialists including gastroenterologist, pediatric surgeon, transplant surgeons, clinical dietitians, and a clinical nurse specialist. Each patient is evaluated with a history and physical examination, review of pertinent laboratory data, and nutritional assessment. Subsequently, a coordinated treatment plan and goals are constructed and implemented for local patients or communicated to local physicians. Since the inception of the ICC center, a total of 389 patients (61% male, 70% Caucasian) have been evaluated with a median age of 1year at referral (range1day to 28.8 years). Median small bowel length was 25 cm. After informed consent was obtained at the time of their initial evaluation, database registry information was recorded for each patient from patient or parental reports, medical records as well as operative and pathology reports. Registry data include demographic information, a baseline physical assessment by systems, intestinal characteristics (including small bowel length, the percent of small bowel remaining after initial surgery, bowel lengthening procedures and the presence/absence of an ileocecal valve and large intestine), anthropometric data, mode of nutrition therapy, and transplant status. The percent of small bowel remaining after initial surgery are estimated using normal values for intestinal length. Follow-up anthropometric and nutrition therapy data are also collected biannually. Disease associated complications including death, graft failure, or the development of micronutrient deficiencies and food allergies, among others, are monitored and recorded. Medical management of the patients who were TPN-dependent resulted in 42 (12%) subsequently being weaned from TPN without further surgical intervention (median time to wean=1.5years). Active patients on TPN who continue to be managed medically (n=23) have advanced from a mean of 88% caloric intake from TPN at referral to 56% currently with a median follow-up time of 2years. Twenty five patients received a bowel lengthening procedure. Of these, 8(32%) successfully weaned from TPN without transplantation and 11proceeded to transplant with the majority subsequently weaning from TPN. The remaining six patients failed to wean from TPN without transplantation. Nucci et al., [18] conclude that the Intestinal Rehabilitation Program at the Children's Hospital of Pittsburgh, which included an aggressive medical and nutritional intervention along with early referral, intestinal lengthening procedures, and intestinal transplantation in children with intestinal failure dependent on parenteral nutrition resulted in the achievement of enteral autonomy and improved survival.

A multidisciplinary IRP formed by a pediatric gastroenterologist, a surgeon, a dietitian, a nurse practitioner, and a nurse coordinator was started at the University of Nebraska Medical Center in October 2000 [19]. Nebraska Medical Center is a referral center and 90% of the patients came from different locations throughout the country. When these patients were enrolled in the IRP, all of them stayed in Omaha for at least the first 2 months after evaluation. The philosophy of the program was to use multiple therapies to promote intestinal adaptation and the eventual weaning of patients off PN. Treatment options for SBS in children include long-term PN, intestinal rehabilitation, and/or intestinal transplantation. Aggressive enteral therapies, along with maintenance of hydration, by trained medical staff were important factors in long-term survival. The components of the IRP in children included: 1)physical, biochemical, radiological, and histological evaluation of patients' condition, identifying the anatomy and possible abnormalities of the intestinal tract; 2) parent/patient education; 3)enteral tube feedings; 4)parenteral nutrition management/weaning; 5) management of complications of intestinal failure (eg, sepsis, catheter-related, bacterial overgrowth); 6) psychosocial support; 7) surgical options to restore intestinal continuity, repair enterocutaneous fistulas, and resect strictured/obstructed bowel, including intestinal lengthening (Bianchi procedure) and serial transverse enteroplasty;

the decision of any surgical options depends on the age, intestinal length, and intestinal anatomy, as well as bowel diameter; 8) investigational pharmacological agent. Torres et al., [19] details the outcomes of children with intestinal failure referred for liver/small bowel transplantation during a 4-year period who, after a complete evaluation, were treated by the IRP. 51 PN-dependent patients with intestinal failure referred for liver/small bowel transplantation were enrolled in the IRP after a complete evaluation. This group's experience with the IRP demonstrates that more aggressive attempts at intestinal rehabilitation are warranted in many patients with SBS who have risk factors previously identified for poor prognosis in terms of total PN weaning or survival. In 75% of these selected patients, Nebraska's team has achieved long-term survival, weaned patients from PN, and avoided the need for long-term immunosuppression. Torres et al., suggests that the success of the program can be related mostly to a comprehensive medical/surgical approach and close follow-up by trained medical staff. The medical treatment of patients in an IRP is focused on an aggressive dietary management with precise control of the metabolic balance, as well as prompt and effective treatment of patient complications. Continual parent education and support is also an important part of the program. The advantage of having a rehabilitation program in a transplant center is that the line between the 2 programs is contiguous, making it possible for a patient to move from 1 program to the other in a timely fashion. The authors conclude that with an aggressive medical and surgical approach, even patients with intestinal failure and advanced liver disease can avoid transplantation. The patients in the IRP at the Nebraska Medical Center showed improved liver function and nutritional parameters with the ability to discontinue PN while maintaining growth. Early referral of patients with intestinal failure to specialized centers before the development of advanced liver disease is recommended.

The Intestinal Rehabilitation Program at the Cleveland Clinic was founded in 2001 to care for patients with intestinal failure. The main goal of the program was to safely reduce or avoid the need for long-term TPN through dietary and medical therapy with referral for surgical reconstruction or small bowel transplantation if indicated [20]. Starting with 3 patients in 2001, the program expanded to evaluate and care for 150 new patients in 2007 and more than 180 new patients in 2008. Assessment of bowel anatomy through operative reports, pathology reports, intestinal imaging, and plasma citrulline level is performed to determine bowel structure and function. Clinical monitoring includes daily urine outputs, daily weight, and presence of thirst. Laboratory monitoring includes weekly measurement of electrolytes along with calcium, phosphorus, magnesium, serum urea nitrogen, and creatinine. A thorough evaluation of the patient's gastrointestinal anatomy, nutrition and hydration status, enteral and parenteral intake, urine and gastrointestinal losses, and the use of antidiarrheal and other medications is performed on initial Intestinal Rehabilitation Program referral and at subsequent intervals. Within 4 to 6 weeks after resection, patients with an enterostomy gradually resume eating fibrous foods and begin soluble fiber supplementation as tolerated to add bulk and prolong transit time through the remaining bowel. Patients unable to consume adequate nutrition orally benefit from enteral nutrition infused at a slow rate into the gastrointestinal tract through a nasogastric feeding tube or a percutaneous endoscopic gastrostomy tube. Home parenteral nutrition was started at the Cleveland Clinic in 1975 and its use has rapidly expanded during the last 37 years. The number of patients who are dis charged by the TPN team exceeds 200 per year. Most patients need TPN for less than 6 months either to manage complicated surgical conditions that resolve spontaneously or to restore gastrointestinal continuity and function through staged procedures. A multidisciplinary hospital-based team evaluates, initiates, and manages patients with home TPN (HPN). After the patient is approved to receive HPN by a nutrition support team physician, an appropriate vascular access device is placed. Every HPN candidate is re-evaluated by a case manager, social worker, nurse, dietitian, and physician before discharge. Before 1997, most patients were completely trained in the hospital for 2 to 3 weeks. Currently, training is initiated in the hospital and completed at home for 2 to 3 days. Interactive and video tape dedicational interventions have been shown to reduce catheter-related blood stream infections, number of hospitalizations, and reactive depression and are currently being updated [21]. Patients are asked to record their weight, fluid intake and output, temperature, and urine dipstick for sugar results daily. Routine laboratory work includes serum complete blood cell count, electrolytes, urea nitrogen, creatinine, glucose, calcium, albumin, liver enzymes, bilirubin, magnesium, and phosphorus. These studies are performed weekly until the results are stable and then monthly. Serum trace elements are checked initially and then every 6 months. Shatnawei and coworkers conclude that establishment of the Intestinal Rehabilitation Program at the Cleveland Clinic allowed to avoid in selected patients the need for long-term parenteral nutrition and reserves intestinal transplantation for children who fail intestinal rehabilitation or are deemed to have no significant chance for enteral feeding tolerance.

The Intestinal Failure Program at Seattle Children's Hospital was formally established in January 2005. Its goal was to function as a regional referral center for all children with intestinal failure regardless of etiology as well as for patients who are being prepared for or who have undergone intestinal transplantation [22]. The program's home institution has a large regional catchment area and serves as the only free standing tertiary-care pediatric institution for a 5-state area and is the only pediatric liver and intestine transplantation program for 6 states. The program was created by experienced clinicians recruited from reputable programs and is a true multidisciplinary collaboration in that every patient is evaluated by pediatric gastroenterologists, pediatric general surgeons, intestinal failure nutritionists, pharmacists with advanced training in parenteral nutrition, and social workers. Transplant gastroenterologists and transplant surgeons see all relevant patients. All patients referred to the Intestinal Failure Program are entered into a prospective database that collects background data and is routinely updated as children continue in the program. This data base is maintained weekly by the program's primary care givers, including nurse practitioners and physicians. During 2005-2008, forty-nine patients were referred to and treated in the Intestinal Failure Program. The median age at referral was 7months. Nineteen patients (39%) originated with in regional institution, and an additional 33% of patients were referred from out of state. In total, 78% of children were referred from within the broader geographic region, which comprises Washington, Wyoming, Alaska, Montana, and Idaho. Thirteen bowel-lengthening procedures were performed, all in the form of the serial transverse enteroplasty procedure. With a median follow-up period of 14 months, the overall survival rate was 88%. Enteral autonomy was achieved in 22 patients (45%). In evaluating the intermediate-term outcomes of intestinal failure patients seen in a new regional referral center at Seattle Children's Hospital, Javid et al., conclude that a new multidisciplinary program for pediatric intestinal failure can grow quickly and develop successful regional outreach beyond its home institution; within 5 years of inception, one third of patients originated from out of state and most children were referred from the contiguous 5-state geographic region. The evolution and success of Seatle's Intestinal Failure program reinforces the concept of highly specialized care concentrated in a central referral institution. Indeed, because the treatment of these children mandates diverse expertise and continues to evolve rapidly, Javid et al., conclude that long-term management of intestinal failure patients should be organized solely at dedicated tertiary-care pediatric centers. The presented data demonstrate that a newly established intestinal failure program can achieve excellent survival in a cohort of chronically ill and complicated children that has historically been associated with substantial mortality.

Conclusion

Multi-disciplinary teams are believed to be the best approach to successful and integrated care. In analyzing, reflecting and reporting on their programs, several studies have reported great subjective benefit since the introduction of an intestinal rehabilitation program. Pediatric Intestinal Failure Consortium, a multidisciplinary collaborative consisting of 14 pediatric hospitals throughout the United States and Canada, has been developed and is implementing prospective, multi-institutional studies to better define the specific aspects of intestinal failure management that optimize long-term out comes. The published data from these studies suggest that intestinal failure in pediatric patients is quite treatable and provide further evidence that all infants at risk for intestinal failure should be treated aggressively and referred early to a dedicated intestinal rehabilitation center. These data also high light the effectiveness of intestinal rehabilitation in the care of these patients, although certain limitations exist. In these clinics, rehabilitation of the gut is prioritized before committing children to solid organ transplantation. The principles of intestinal rehabilitation followed in these programs include early restoration of intestinal continuity, the liberal use of continuous gastrostomy feedings, administration of hypocaloric elemental formulas to optimize enterocyte absorption, use of operative bowel-lengthening techniques in dilated bowel, and aggressive antibiotic treatment of bacterial over-growth. These data indicate that intestinal rehabilitation alone is associated with successful enteral feeding advancement, improved liver function, and an excellent survival rate, although many of these patients remain at least partially dependent on provisions of parenteral nutrition. These patients are at risk for progressive liver disease, and longer term data are required to better substantiate the advantages of intestinal rehabilitation.

References

[1] Vanderhoof, JA. Short bowel syndrome. *Neonat Gastroenterol*, 1996, 23, 377.

[2] Booth, IW; Lander AD: Short bowel syndrome. *Bailliere's Clin Gastroenterol*, 1998, 12, 739.

[3] Sigalet, DL. Short bowel syndrome in infants and children: an overview. *Semin Pediatr Surg*, 2001, 10, 49.

[4] Chaet, MS; Farrell, MK; Ziegler, MM; Warner, BW. Intensive nutritional support and remedial surgical intervention for extreme short bowel syndrome. *Pediat Gastroenterol Nutr*, 1994, 19, 295.
[5] DiBaise, JK; Young, RJ; Vanderhoof, JA. Intestinal rehabilitation and the short bowel syndrome. *Am J Gastroenterol*, 2004, 99, 1386.
[6] Sturm, A; Layer, P; Goebell, H. Short-bowel syndrome: an update on the therapeutic approach. *Scand J Gastroenterol*, 1997, 32, 289.
[7] Thompson, JS. Inflammatory disease and outcome of short bowel syndrome. *Am J Surg*, 2000, 180, 551.
[8] Coran, AG; Spivak, D; Teitelbaum, DH. An analysis of the morbidity and mortality of short bowel syndrome in the pediatric age group. *Eur J Pediatr Surg*, 1999, 9,228.
[9] Mayr, JM; Schober, PH; Weißensteiner, U; Höllwarth, ME. Morbidity and mortality of the short bowel syndrome. *Eur J Pediatr Surg*, 1999, 9, 231.
[10] Spencer, AU; Neaga, A; West, B; Safran, J; Brown, P; Btaiche, I. Pediatric short bowel syndrome redefining predictors of success. *Ann Surg*, 2005, 242, 403.
[11] Chaet, MS; Farrell, MK; Ziegler, MM; Warner, BW. Intensive nutritional support and remedial surgical intervention for extreme short bowel syndrome. *Pediatr Gastroenterol Nutr*, 1994, 19, 295.
[12] Goulet, O; Baglin-Gobet, S; Jais, JP; Michel, JL; Jan, D; Ricour, C. Outcome and long-term growth after extensive small bowel resection in the neonatal period: a survey of 87 children. *Eur J Pediatr Surg*, 2005, 15, 95.
[13] Guarino, A; De Marco, G. Italian National Network for Pediatric Intestinal Failure. Natural history of intestinal failure, investigated through a national network-based approach. *J Pediatr Gastroenterol Nutr*, 2003, 37, 136–141.
[14] Koehler, AN; Yaworski, JA; Gardner, M. Coordinated interdisciplinary management of pediatric intestinal failure: a 2-year review. *J Pediatr Surg*, 2000, 35, 380.
[15] Goulet, O; Ruemmele, F; Lacaille, F; Colomb, V. Irreversible intestinal failure. *J Pediatr Gastroenterol Nutr*, 2004, 38, 250.
[16] Fishbein, TM; Schiano, T; LeLeiko, N. An integrated approach to intestinal failure: results of a new program with total parenteral nutrition, bowel rehabilitation, and transplantation. *J Gastrointest Surg*, 2002, 6, 554.

[17] Dudrick, SJ; O'Donnell, JJ; Englert, DM; Matheny, RG; Blume, ER; Nutt, RE; Hickey, MS; Barroso, AO. 100 patient-years of ambulatory home total parenteral nutrition. *Ann Surg*, 1984, 199, 770.

[18] Nucci, A; Burns, RC; Armah, T; Lowery, c; Yaworski, JA; Strohm, S; Bond, G; Mazariegos, G; Squires, R. Interdisciplinary Management of Pediatric Intestinal Failure: A 10-year Review of Rehabilitation and Transplantation. *J Gastrointest Surg*, 2008, 12, 429.

[19] Torres, C; Sudan, D; Vanderhoof, J; Grant, W; Botha, J; Raynor, S; Langnas, A. Role of an intestinal rehabilitation program in the treatment of advanced intestinal failure. *J Pediatr Gastroenterol Nutr.*, 2007, 45, 204.

[20] Shatnawei, A; Parekh, NR; Rhoda, KM; Speerhas, R; Stafford, J; Dasari, V; Quintini, C; Kirby, DF; Steiger, E. Intestinal Failure Management at the Cleveland Clinic. *Arch Surg*, 2010, 145, 521.

[21] Grischkan, D; Steiger, E; Fazio, V. Maintenance of home hyperalimentation in patients with high-output jejunostomies. *Arch Surg*, 1979, 114, 838.

[22] Javid, PJ; Malone, FR; Reyes, J; Healey, PJ; Horslen, SP. The experience of a regional pediatric intestinal failure program: Successful outcomes from intestinal rehabilitation. *Am J Surg*, 2010, 199, 676.

In: Short Bowel Syndrome in Children
Editor: Igor Sukhotnik
ISBN: 978-1-62948-518-8

Chapter IX

Bowel-Preserving Surgery for Short Bowel Syndrome

Yechiel Sweed, M.D.*

Department of Pediatric Surgery, Nahariya Medical Center,
Nahariya and Faculty of Medicine in the Galilee,
Bar Ilan University, Safed, Israel

Abstract

Short Bowel Syndrome (SBS) results in loss of absorptive capacity in the gut, leading to malabsorption due to protein, energy, fluid and electrolyte loss and imbalance while on the enteral diet alone. Various non-surgical and surgical therapeutic options have emerged that have improved the survival outcome following SBS in both children and adults. An individualized complex, multi-disciplinary approach to medical and surgical rehabilitation is needed to provide an opportunity for enteral autonomy to be possible in a patient with SBS. Multiple surgical techniques are available to address the patient with SBS. The two most commonly applied techniques are those labeled as intestinal lengthening procedures. These include the LILT (Longitudinal Intestinal Lengthening) described by Bianchi and the more recent STEP (Serial

* Address correspondence to Sweed Y, MD: Dept of Pediatric Surgery, Nahariya Medical Center, Faculty of Medicine in the Galilee, Bar Ilan University, Safed, Israel. E-mail: yechiel.sweed@naharia.health.gov.il.

Transverse Enteroplasty) described by Kim. These "lengthening" procedures correct bacterial overgrowth by correcting the dilatation and dysmotility, leading to improved absorption and a decreased need for bowel transplantation. The remnant bowel of the patient with SBS plays a very pivotal role in autologous gastrointestinal reconstruction (AGIR) surgery. Intestinal transplantation should be reserved for patients with failed AGIR or those who have no prospect for autologous enteral autonomy.

Keywords: Short bowel syndrome, Intestinal failure, LILT (longitudinal Intestinal Lengthening), STEP (Serial Transverse Enteroplasty), AGIR (Autologous Gastrointestinal Reconstruction), PN (Parenteral Nutrition)

Bowel Adaptation

Intestinal failure resulting from loss of intestinal length can be devastating at any age. Following massive bowel resection and a loss of enterocyte mass, malabsorption occurs due to both decreased contact of the nutrients with the mucosa and decreased intestinal transit time. After bowel resection there is "adaptation" of the bowel remnant which is sufficient in some patients, especially those with limited resection, to support growth and long term survival.

With normal bowel adaptation, both micro – and macroscopic changes occur within the intestine, which lead to smooth muscle hypertrophy, increases in villus height and crypt depth, proliferation of enterocytes and macroscopic bowel dilatation. Adaptation occurs rapidly during the initial 4-24 months, then becomes slower and plateaus over several years [1,2]. In some patients, however, bowel adaptation leads to excessive dilatation with disordered motility, resulting in stasis, bacterial overgrowth and decreased absorption of nutrients. Bacterial translocation from this dilated dysmotile gut activates production of nitric oxide or cytokines such as tumor necrosis factor which is hypothesized to ultimately lead to liver injury [3].

Autologous gastrointestinal reconstruction (AGIR) is a term used to describe surgical intervention to restore intestinal function. AGIR can serve to correct the stasis and bacterial overgrowth, as well as increase transit time, thereby correcting the dilatation and motility disorder and increasing mucosal absorption [4]. In many patients AGIR may be a definitive therapy to achieve enteral autonomy. In others, there is improvement in the overall medical condition to allow the patient to become a bowel transplant candidate.

1. Causes of SBS and Surgical Strategy in the Neonate

The surgical treatment options for neonatal SBS include bowel conservation at the time of initial presentation, bowel lengthening operations and intestinal transplantation.

Bowel conservation has an important role in the prevention of SBS, and treatment of patients who develop SBS. The causes of neonatal and pediatric SBS include necrotizing enterocolitis (NEC), intestinal atresia, gastroschisis, malrotation and volvulus, and Hirschsprung's disease. The most common cause is NEC. The incidence of NEC is highly dependent upon birth weight, with those neonates between 500-750 grams, having a 12% incidence of NEC [5]. In NEC the prime predictor of eventual intestinal failure remains residual small bowel length [6]. A neonate with surgical NEC may have SBS secondary to small intestinal loss compounded by malabsorption and disordered motility, as a result of damaged viable bowel that has remained in situ. In practice the terms intestinal failure and SBS are often used interchangeably.

In the absence of any surgical bowel lengthening and tapering procedures, 35 cm of neonatal small bowel is associated with a 50% probability of weaning from parenteral nutrition (PN) [7]. However a relatively wide variance is evident and patients with much longer bowel lengths sometimes do not wean from PN. Poor motility and/or ischemic injury incurred to the remaining bowel may contribute to this finding. Conversely, neonates with as little as 10 cm of residual small intestine can sometimes be weaned from PN. It is important to emphasize that the more premature the neonate the more likely the intestine will grow in length subsequently [4]. Generally, premature neonates have a greater capacity than full term infants for intestinal growth, and hence bowel adaptation. Nonetheless, residual neonatal small intestinal length remains the single major positive clinical predictor of ultimate enteral feeding tolerance [6,7].

The initial surgical operation is aimed at limiting as much bowel loss as possible. In patients undergoing surgery for NEC where the viability of the bowel is in question, the use of a 'second look' operation within 24 hours may be employed. With this approach marginally viable intestine is left in situ, the patient is resuscitated and the bowel is then reassessed at second operation. Only the clearly necrotic intestine is then excised [4]. The use of a temporary transparent plastic 'silo' to cover the bowel is sometimes also helpful to avoid the risk of inducing abdominal compartment syndrome. Once bowel edema has subsided delayed abdominal closure can be accomplished.

The prompt establishment of bowel continuity through stomal closure is associated with more rapid weaning from PN [7]. Usually the surgeon will wait approximately 6 weeks between operations in an effort to minimize the vascularity of any adhesions that may have formed. In cases where the neonate is unstable, the time of surgery may be further delayed. Careful discussions between the surgeon, neonatologist and anesthesiologist are mandatory when considering the timing of surgery in ill SBS patients [4].

In a neonate born with intestinal atresia and limited distal small intestine (usually < 35cm), tapering of the dilated segment, or tapering and lengthening either by Bianchi procedure [8,9] or by a primary STEP enteroplasty [10] may be done.

2. Autologous Intestinal Reconstruction

Up to 75% of patients with SBS will eventually achieve PN independence [11]. The remaining 25% may fail to adapt because of dysmotility, bacterial overgrowth or very short residual small intestinal length. Autologous bowel reconstruction may prove beneficial for this subgroup of patients [12-17].

Timing of Surgical Intervention

The time of surgical intervention is very important. One does not want to intervene too early when the patient has capacity to adapt independently, but if surgery is delayed too long, irreversible intestinal failure associated liver disease (IFALD) may develop, and then transplantation becomes the appropriate intervention. The recommended strategy is to wait until the patients plateau in their enteral tolerance, and they are unable to further wean the PN.

A patient who begins to develop complications such as bacterial overgrowth, recurrent sepsis or IFALD becomes a candidate for autologous reconstruction [18]. The choice of procedure is dependent on the baseline functional capacity of the intestine, the intestinal caliber and the residual length of bowel.

Surgical Therapy

There are multiple strategies for surgical therapy for SBS (Table 1). They may be divided into strategies restoring intestinal continuity (takedown enterostomy), relieving obstruction and dysmotility (strictureplasty or bowel tapering for dilated bowel segments) and lengthening the remaining dilated intestine (Bianchi procedure or serial transverse enteroplasty - STEP). Other strategies include prolonging transit time, (reversed intestinal segments, colonic interposition or creation of artificial sphincters), or transplanting new intestine [17].

Table 1. Transplant and non-transplant surgical options to treat SBS

Aim of Procedure	To improve peristalsis	To increase passage time	To increase absorptive surface area
Procedure	Tapering	Antiperistaltic segment	Serosal patching
	Tapering and lengthening	Colon interposition	Mucosal transplantation
		Intestinal valves	Small bowel intestinal transplantation
		Artificial invagination	

3. Inefficient Peristalsis - Surgical Procedures

Tapering

Tapering of dilated loops can be accomplished by a triangular resection of an antimesenteric bowel wall (Figure 1a). The disadvantage of this type of tapering is that it reduces the available intestinal surface area. Thus, the technique can be reserved for short segments or when intestinal lengthening procedures are not applicable.

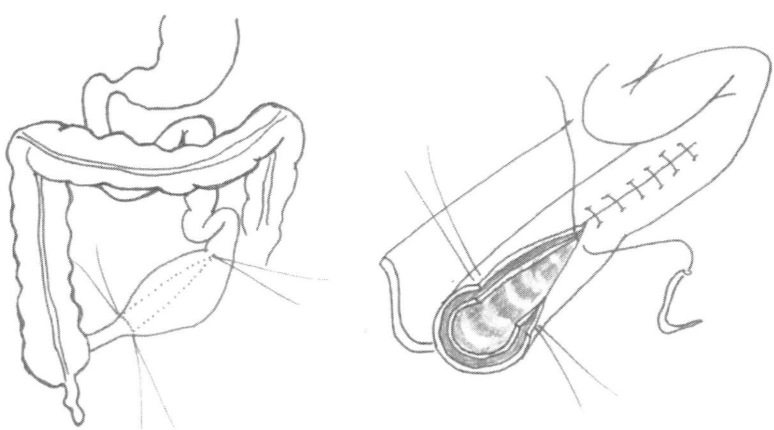

Figure 1a. Tapering is performed by resection of a triangular antimesenteric bowel wall.

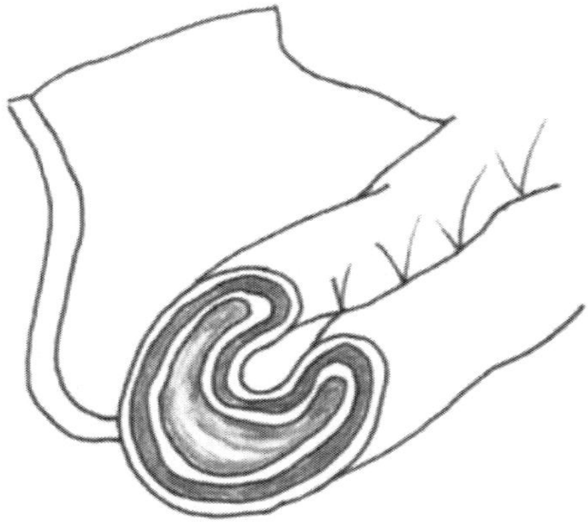

Figure 1b. Tapering is done by turning in the redundant tissue. This approach saves all the available absorptive surface area.

Intestinal tapering was introduced by Howard and Othersen [19], in a short segment of dilated bowel with disordered motility causing intestinal stasis. Grosfeld et al [20] later modified this technique using a stapler to perform resection of the redundant antimesenteric bowel wall.

Tapering can also be accomplished simply by turning in the redundant antimesenteric bowel wall (Figure 1b). This technique, which was reported by De Lorimier and Harrison [21], avoids reduction of intestinal surface area while preserving enterocyte mass and results in improvement of bowel function [22-24]. However, although initially successful, the suture line that holds the plication in place occasionally breaks down, which allows the bowel to unravel into its former dilated and poorly mobile state.

4. Intestinal Lengthening Operations

A. Longitudinal Intestinal Lengthening and Tailoring Operation (LILT)

The Longitudinal Intestinal Lengthening and Tailoring operation (LILT) was introduced by Bianchi in 1980 [8,9]. This ingenious but technically challenging operation utilized the concept that dilated small intestine is supplied by 2 separate leaves of mesentery [Fig 2]. The Bianchi bowel lengthening procedure was first applied clinically by Baeckman and Taylor

[25] in 1981 to a 4-year old boy who had SBS secondary to gastroschisis and intrauterine volvulus.

The child was PN dependent with a 50 cm jejunum and was also at risk from precarious venous access. Within 10 weeks after surgery, the patient was able to wean off PN and has continued to thrive on enteral nutrition.

The procedure consisting of longitudinal deviation of the dilated part into 2 separate segments each comprising one half of the circumference (Figure 2). Both segments remain viable because the mesenteric vessels are divided carefully extramurally into branches separately supplying either side of the bowel. The two halves are then refashioned into tubes of normal intestinal diameter which are lined up in an isoperistaltic manner and anastomosed one to the other yielding twice the length of the original part. Propulsion, although not uniform is effectively isoperistaltic with a reduction in stasis and sepsis. The slower transit and longer mucosal contact enhances adaptively and improves absorption.

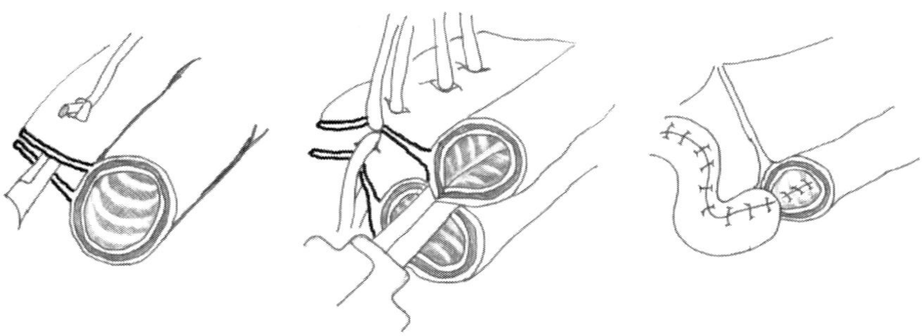

Figure 2. Bianchi's Tapering and Lengthening procedure.

Post-operative complications producing moderate morbidity have been reported; these include stenosis at the hemi-loop anastomosis, inter-loop fistula, loss of hemi-loop from vascular compromise and recurrent dilatation [26,27]. Bianchi reviewed the worldwide experience with LILT in 2006. He reported on 150 patients from 8 published studies and found overall survival ranging from 30%-100%, and ability to wean from PN ranging widely from 28-100% [9]. Several series worldwide have reported their results using the LILT procedure [28-31]. Waag et al [28] reported 6 year follow-up of 25 patients who underwent LILT. Of the 18 survivors, 17 were able to be weaned from PN and there were no intraoperative deaths. King et al [31] reported on their systematic literature review of Bianchi and STEP procedures, and found that the overall survival for the last 15 years has been 89% with no significant difference between the two procedures. They also reported that the Bianchi procedure has a higher rate of weaning patients who were static on parenteral nutrition with conservative measures: 55% vs. 48%. However the Bianchi procedure was associated with a higher rate of patients receiving transplantations: 10% vs. 6 %.

B. Serial Transverse Entheroplasty (STEP) Procedure

The latest addition to the AGIR technique has been the STEP procedure introduced by Kim et al in 2003 [13]. The technique was first described in a porcine model with studies reporting a 68% increase in bowel length post procedure. Later in the same year, Kim et al [14] preformed the first human STEP procedure in a two year old child with gastroschisis who had previously undergone a LILT procedure. STEP was applied to a 83 cm-long dilated small bowel, increasing the length to 147 cm.

The STEP technique (Fig 3) uses a stapler applied perpendicularly to the long axis of the bowel to partially transect the intestine. Each staple firing begins from alternating sides so that the bowel is divided transversely at equidistant intervals, leading to a final diameter of approximately 2cm. The zigzag bowel pattern created at the end of the procedure appears to straighten out in most patients over a period of time. The salient advantages of this operation are that it is technically straightforward, it results in a uniform bowel channel regardless of variable underlying bowel dilation, and it can be repeated subsequently if bowel becomes redilated [32]. Animal studies have shown that the STEP is associated with improved nutrient absorption, enhanced growth and overall increase in bowel surface area as reflected by elevated citrulin levels [33].

The STEP operation has been performed successfully and safely in many centers around the world [34,35,36]. Recently, Jones et al reported on 111 consecutive patients enrolled in the international STEP data registry [10]. They found that the overall mortality post STEP for the first 15 years was 11% and that the pre-STEP factors for progressing to transplantation or death were higher direct bilirubin and shorter bowel length. They also reported that 47% of the group attained full enteral nutrition post-STEP and that patients with longer pre-STEP bowel length were significantly more likely to achieve enteral autonomy.

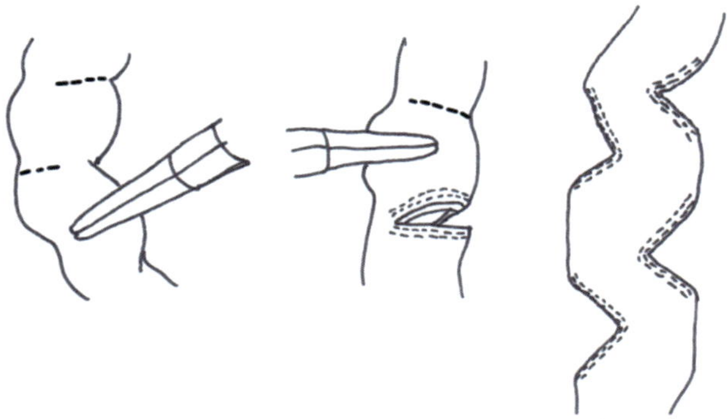

Figure 3. Serial Transverse Enteroplasty (STEP) procedure.

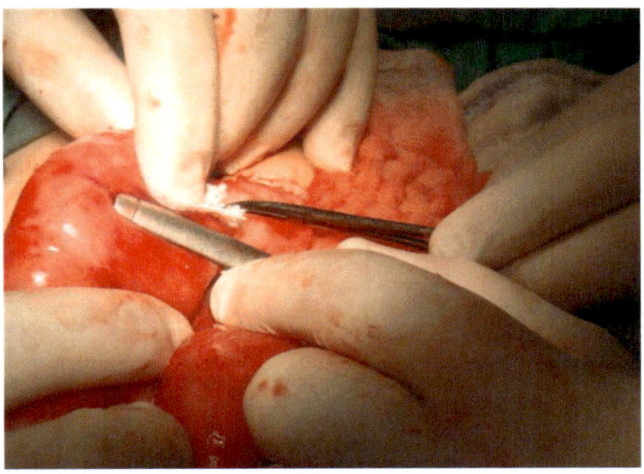

9(a)

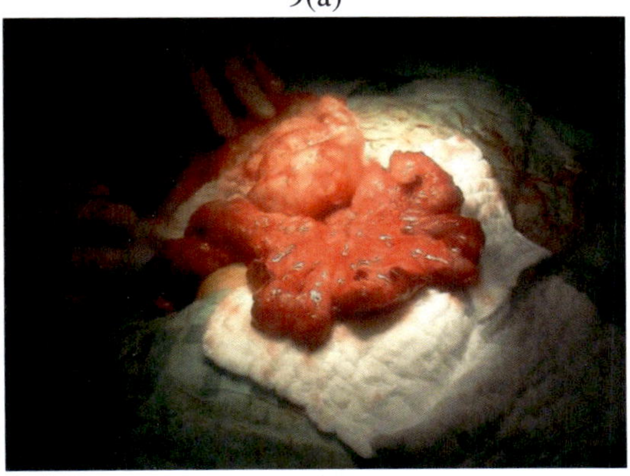

9(b)

Picture 9(a) and 9(b). (a) Stapler positioned at the mesenteric border of the bowel. (b) After completion of the STEP procedure.

5. Procedures for Prolonged Intestinal Transit Time

There are three surgical procedures designed to prolong intestinal transit time which have been evaluated. These include anti-peristaltic segment, colonic interposition, intestinal valves and artificial invagination. The anti-peristaltic segment technique is the most common procedure of those reported.

Reversed Intestinal Segment

Reversing a segment of intestine to slow intestinal transit has been studied experimentally for many years. Gibson et al [37] reported the first use of reversal of small intestine in an adult. Since then this surgical procedure has been a commonly used method for patients with SBS (Figure 4).

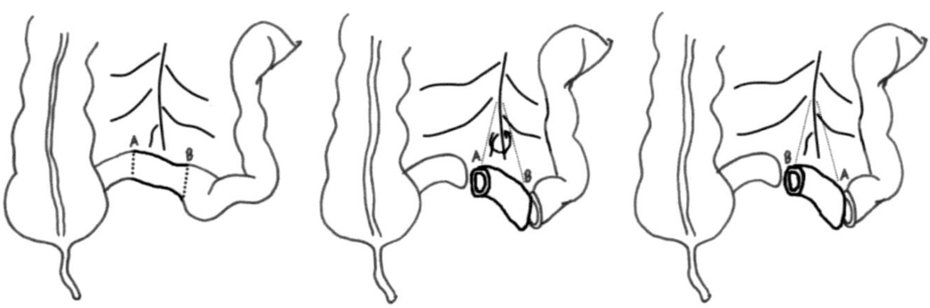

Figure 4. Antiperistaltic segment.

The anti-peristaltic small bowel segment functions as a physiological valve by causing retrograde peristalsis, and therefore it should always be located at the end of small intestinal remnant to receive the benefit of the proximal absorptive surface. Most experimental studies of antiperistalsis segments demonstrate slowed intestinal transit, improved absorption, reduced weight loss and prolonged survival [38,39].

The optimal length of the reversed segment would appear to be approximately 10 cm among adults and 3 cm among children [37,40].Care must be taken to avoid complete rotation of the mesentery to avoid ischemia. Anti-peristaltic segments have been reported clinically in more than 160 patients, of whom approximately 90% were adults [41-43]. Clinical improvement has been reported in 80% of SBS patients. These reports demonstrated slower intestinal transit time and increased absorptive capacity.

Reversed small intestinal segment was used successfully in a 3-month-old patient with SBS who had total of 11 cm of small bowel at the time of surgery [44].

Recently, Beyer–Berjot et al [43] reported on the results of segmental reversal procedure in 38 adult patients with SBS. They found that the reversal procedure has a role as conservative alternative to small bowel transplantation in patients with SBS, permanently dependent on PN. They used a segment of 10-12 cm and reported that almost half the patients can be weaned from PN.

Colonic Interposition

Isoperistaltic or antiperistaltic interposition of colon has the advantage of using none of the small intestinal remnants (Figure 5). The method was developed by Hutcher et al [45,46]. The isoperistaltic segment should be interposed proximally either between the jejunum and ileum if the jejunal segment is short and the ileal segment long, or between the duodenum and jejunum if the latter is long and the ileum short. Isoperistaltic colonic interposition slows down the rate at which nutrients are delivered to the distal intestine by slowing peristalsis. Panis et al [42] reported a success rate of 50% with colonic transposition among patients with SBS, and also suggested that isoperistaltic transposition may be better than antiperistaltic.

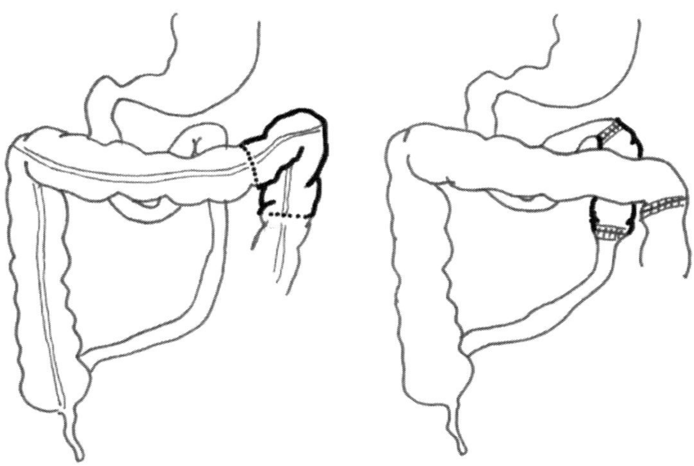

Figure 5. Isoperistaltic interposition of colon.

The optimal length of an interposed colon has not yet been defined. Glick et al [48] used 10-15 cm segments in small babies, while Garcia et al [49] used a 24 cm segment in a 14 month old infant.

A reversed colonic interposition primarily causes a potential functional obstruction by delaying the emptying of the proximal bowel. It should therefore always be located distally to the small bowel remnant [50]. The interposed colonic segment adapts to the function of the small bowel and can absorb water, electrolytes and nutrient by active transport mechanism [51]. Reported clinical results show that out of seven infants with isoperistaltic interposition, four survived [48-49].

An adult patient with 5 cm of jejunum and 7 cm of ileum after a midgut volvulus could be weaned from PN completely by an 18 cm segment of isoperistaltic colon [52].

Reference

[1] Goulet O, Ruemmele F, Lacaille F. Irreversible intestinal failure. *J. Pediatr. Gastroenterol. Nutr.* 2004;38:250-69.

[2] Barksdale EM, Stanford A. The surgical management of short bowel syndrome. *Curr. Gastroenterol. Rep.* 2002;4:229-37.

[3] Shiomi M, Wakabayashi Y, Sano T. Nitric oxide suppression reversibly attenuates mitochondrial dysfunction and cholestasis in endotoxemic rat liver. *Hepatology* 1998;27:108-115.

[4] Gutierrez IM, Kang KH, Jaksic T, Neonatal short bowel syndrome, Seminars in Fetal & Neonatal Medicine 2011;16: 157-63.

[5] Fitzgibbons SC, Ching Y, Yu D, Carpenter J. Mortality of necrotizing enterocolitis expressed by birth weight categories. *J. Pediatr. Surg.* 2009; 44:1072-5.

[6] Duro D, Kalish LA, Johnston P. Risk factors for intestinal failure in infants with necrotizing enterocolitis: a Glaser Pediatric Research Network study. *J. Pediatr.* 2010; 157:203-8.

[7] Andorsky DJ, Lund DP, Lillehei CW. Nutritional and other postoperative management of neonates with short bowel syndrome correlates with clinical outcomes. *J. Pediatr.* 2001; 139:27-33.

[8] Bianchi A, Intestinal loop lengthening--a technique for increasing small intestinal length. *J. Pediat.r Surg*. 1980;15:145-51.

[9] Bianchi A. From the cradle to enteral autonomy: the role of autologous gastrointestinal reconstruction. *Gastroenterology* 2006; 130: 138-46.
[10] Jones BA, Hull MA, Potanos KM. Report of 111 consecutive patients enrolled in the International Serial Transverse Enteroplasty (STEP) Data Registry: a retrospective observational study. *J. Am. Coll. Surg.* 2013; 216:438-46.
[11] O'Brien DP, Nelson LA, Huang FS. Intestinal adaptation: structure, function, and regulation. *Semin. Pediatr. Surg.* 2001; 10:56-64.
[12] Ching YA, Fitzgibbons S, Valim C. Long-term nutritional and clinical outcomes after serial transverse enteroplasty at a single institution. *J. Pediatr. Surg.* 2009; 44:939-43.
[13] Kim HB, Fauza D, Garza J. Serial transverse enteroplasty (STEP): a novel bowel lengthening procedure. *J. Pediatr. Surg.* 2003; 38:425-9.
[14] Kim HB, Lee PW, Garza J, et al. Serial transverse enteroplasty for short bowel syndrome: a case report. *J. Pediatr. Surg.* 2003;38:881-5.
[15] Javid PJ, Sanchez SE, Horslen SP. Intestinal lengthening and nutritional outcomes in children with short bowel syndrome. *Am. J. Surg.* 2013; 205:576-80.
[16] Pakarinen MP, Kurvinan A, Koivualo AI. Long-term controlled outcomes after autologous intestinal reconstruction surgery in treatment of severe short bowel syndrome. *J. Pediatr. Surg.* 2013;48:339-44.
[17] Sudan D, Thompson J, Botha J. Comparison of intestinal lengthening procedures for patients with short bowel syndrome. *Ann. Surg.* 2007; 246:593-601.
[18] Oliveira C, de Silva N, Wales PW. Five-year outcomes after serial transverse enteroplasty in children with short bowel syndrome. *J. Pediatr. Surg.* 2012; 47(5):931-7.
[19] Howard ER, Othersen HB Jr. Proximal jejunoplasty in the treatment of jejunal atresia. *J. Pediatr. Surg.* 1973; 8:685-90.
[20] Grosfeld JL, Ballantine TVN, Shoemaker R. Operative management of intestinal atresia and stenosis based on pathologic findings. *J. Pediatr. Surg.* 1979, 368-75.
[21] de Lorimier AA, Harrison MR. Intestinal plication in the treatment of atresia. *J. Pediatr. Surg.* 1983;18:734-7.
[22] Thomas CG Jr. Jejunoplasty for the correction of jejunal atresia, *Surg. Gynecol. Obstet.* 1969;129:545-6.
[23] Weber TR, Vane DW, Grosfeld JL. Tapering enteroplasty in infants with bowel atresia and short gut. *Arch. Surg.* 1982;117:684-8.

[24] Ramanujan TM. Functional capability of blind small loops after intestinal remodelling techniques. *Aust. NZ J. Surg.* 1986; 54: 145-50.
[25] Boeckman CR, Traylor R. Bowel lengthening for short gut syndrome. *J. Pediatr. Surg.* 1981;16:996-7.
[26] Thompson JS, Pinch LW, Murray N. Experience with intestinal lengthening for the short-bowel syndrome. *J. Pediatr. Surg.* 1991 ;26:721-4.
[27] Walker SR, Nucci A, Yaworski JA. The Bianchi procedure: a 20-year single institution experience. *J. Pediatr. Surg.* 2006;41:113-9.
[28] Waag KL, Hosie S, Wessel L, What do children look like after longitudinal intestinal lengthening. *Eur. J. Pediatr. Surg.* 1999;9:260-2.
[29] Thompson JS, Pinch LW, Young R. Long-term outcome of intestinal lengthening. *Transplant. Proc.* 2000;32:1242-3.
[30] Hosie S, Loff S, Wirth H. Experience of 49 longitudinal intestinal lengthening procedures for short bowel syndrome. *Eur. J. Pediatr. Surg.* 2006;16:171-5.
[31] King B, Carlson G, Khalil BA. Intestinal bowel lengthening in children with short bowel syndrome: systematic review of the Bianchi and STEP procedures. *World J. Surg.* 2013;37:694-704.
[32] Piper H, Modi BP, Kim HB. The second STEP: the feasibility of repeat serial transverse enteroplasty. *J. Pediatr. Surg.* 2006;41:1951-6.
[33] Chang RW, Javid PJ, Oh JT. Serial transverse enteroplasty enhances intestinal function in a model of short bowel syndrome. *Ann. Surg.* 2006;243:223-8.
[34] Modi BP, Javid PJ, Jaksic T. First report of the international serial transverse enteroplasty data registry: indications, efficacy, and complications. *J. Am. Coll. Surg.* 2007;204:365-71.
[35] Rege AS, Sudan DL, Autologous gastrointestinal reconstruction, Review of the optimal nontransplant surgical options for adults and children with Short Bowel Syndrome. *Nutr. Clin. Pract.* 2013; 28:65-74.
[36] Andres AM, Thompson J, Grant W. Repeat surgical bowel lengthening with the STEP procedure, *Transplantation*;2008,85:1294-99.
[37] Gibson LD, Carter R, Hinshaw DB. Segmental reversal of small intestine after massive bowel resection. Successful case with follow-up examination. *JAMA* 1962;182:952-4.
[38] Digalakis M, Papamichail M, Glava C. Interposition of a reversed jejunal segment enhances intestinal adaptation in short bowel syndrome: an experimental study on pigs. *J. Surg. Res.* 2011;171:551-7.

[39] Kozlowski D , Lescut D , Gambiez L. Surgically reversed small bowel segment in Crohn's disease. *Gastroenterology* 1999;116: A688.

[40] Thompson JS, Rikkers LF, Surgical alternatives for the short bowel syndrome. *Am. J. Gastroenterol.* 1987 ;82:97-106.

[41] Thompson JS, Langnas AN, Pinch LW. Surgical approach to short-bowel syndrome. Experience in a population of 160 patients. *Ann. Surg.* 1995; 222: 600-7.

[42] Y Panis, B Messing, P Rivet. Segmental reversal of the small bowel as an alternative to intestinal transplantation in patients with short bowel syndrome. *Ann. Surg.* 1997; 225: 401-7.

[43] Beyer-Berjot L, Joly F, Maggiori L. Segmental reversal of the small bowel can end permanent parenteral nutrition dependency: an experience of 38 adults with short bowel syndrome. *Ann. Surg.* 2012;256:739-44.

[44] Kurz R, Sauer H. Treatment and metabolic findings in extreme short-bowel syndrome with 11 cm jejunal remnant. *J. Pediatr. Surg.* 1983;18:257-63.

[45] Hutcher NE, Salzberg AM. Pre-ileal transposition of colon to prevent the development of short bowel syndrome in puppies with 90 percent small intestinal resection. *Surgery* 1971;70:189-97.

[46] Hutcher NE, Mendez-Picon G, Salzberg AM. Prejejunal transposition of colon to prevent the development of short bowel syndrome in puppies with 90 per cent small intestine resection. *J. Pediatr. Surg.* 1973;8: 771-7.

[47] Lloyd DA. Antiperistaltic colonic interposition following massive small bowel resection in rats. *J. Pediatr. Surg.* 1981;16:64-9.

[48] Glick PL, de Lorimier AA, Adzick NS. Colon interposition: an adjuvant operation for short-gut syndrome. *J. Pediatr. Surg.* 1984;19:719-25.

[49] Garcia VF, Templeton JM, Eichelberger MR. Colon interposition for the short bowel syndrome. *J. Pediatr. Surg.* 1981;16:994-5.

[50] Höllwarth ME, Short Bowel Syndrome and surgical technique for the baby with short intestines, Ch 66, p 606-614, Newborn Surgery 3rd ed., 2011, Editor Prem Puri.

[51] Sidhu GS, Narasimharao KL, Rani VU. Morphological and functional changes in the gut after massive small bowel resection and colon interposition in rhesus monkeys. *Digestion* 1984; 29:47-54.

[52] Brolin RE. Colon interposition for extreme short bowel syndrome: a case report. *Surgery* 1986;100:576-80.

In: Short Bowel Syndrome in Children
Editor: Igor Sukhotnik

ISBN: 978-1-62948-518-8

Chapter X

Intestine Transplantation in Children

***K. Thacker, FRACP*[1] *and Y. Avitzur, M.D.*[1,2*]**

[1]Division of Gastroenterology, Hepatology and Nutrition
[2]Transplant Centre, Hospital for Sick Children, Toronto, Canada

Abstract

Intestine transplantation (IT) is the recommended therapy for children with intestinal failure and severe complications secondary to parenteral nutrition use. Mortality while waiting for transplantation is higher compared to other solid organ transplantation thus early referral for assessment is critical for an improved outcome. A careful risk assessment is required for continual medical therapy by an experienced team before the decision on listing for IT. Varieties of surgical techniques are available and tailored according to the patient's needs, ranging from isolated intestine to liver-intestine and multivisceral transplantation. Induction with lymphocyte depleting agents followed by maintenance with tacrolimus and steroid based therapy are common immunosuppressive regimens. Despite these regimens up to half of

[*] Corresponding author: Yaron Avitzur MD, Division of Gastroenterology, Hepatology and Nutrition, The Hospital for Sick children, 555 University Ave, Toronto, ON, Canada M5G 1X8, Phone – 416-813-7734, Fax – 416-813-4972, E-mail – yaron.avitzur@sickkids.ca.

all patients experience acute rejection in the early post operative period. Other common complications that might lead to a significant mortality and morbidity include viral, bacterial and fungal infections, post transplant lymphoproliferative disorder, graft vs. host disease, chronic rejection and renal insufficiency. Short-term outcome of patients with IT has seen significant improvements in the last decade. Best results are reported from high volume centers with 3-year survival reaching 70%-84% however only modest improvements in patient and graft survival beyond 5 years after IT limit the long term outcome of IT survivors.

Introduction

Intestine transplantation (IT) remains the recommended therapy for intestinal failure (IF) patients with life threatening complications on parenteral nutrition (PN). IT has evolved and progressed over the last five decades since the first description of IT on an experimental basis by Starzl in 1960[1]. During the pre-Calcineurine era i.e. before 1980 IT was not a viable option due to high rate of severe rejection and graft failure[2, 3]. But overtime several factors led towards the establishment of IT as a standard and successful therapy for IF patients: introduction of Calcineurine inhibitors, better understanding of the pathophysiology and immunology of IT, improved surgical techniques with accumulation of surgical experience and improved methods to monitor and prevent viral infections (Epstein Barr Virus (EBV) and Cytomegalovirus (CMV)). In parallel to the improved outcome after IT major advances in the management of chronic intestinal failure in the past decade has led to significant reduction in the mortality and morbidity associated with PN therapy [4-6] and to a reduction in the need for IT as was recently reported by the International intestinal transplant registry. This chapter will review the indications, surgical techniques, treatment strategies, complications and the outcome of IT.

Referral and Listing Criteria

IF is defined as a reduction of functional gut mass below the minimal amount necessary for digestion and absorption that is adequate to satisfy the nutrient and fluid requirements for growth in children.[7] The causes of IF in children can be divided into 3 categories: loss of gut mass (anatomical – short bowel syndrome), neuromuscular disorders (Chronic intestinal pseudo-obstruction syndromes or intestinal aganglionosis) and intestinal epithelial disorders[7]. Approximately 10% of children with IF will need either isolated IT or IT associated with other organs (liver/multivisceral) despite optimization of their medical and surgical management [7]. The most common causes of IF that lead to IT as reported by the intestinal transplant registry in 2011 are short gut syndrome (68%) with gastroschisis, volvulus and necrotizing enterocolitis as the most common reasons, motility disorders (14%), mucosal defects such as microvillus inclusion disease and tufting enteropathy (10%) and re-transplantation (5%).

Early and timely referral for transplant assessment is critical for improved patient survival while on the transplant waiting list and following transplantation, [8]. High incidence of mortality before IT have been reported in late referrals of patients for pre-transplant assessment, in very young patients due to scarcity of size-matched donors and due to allocation criteria that do not account unique risk factors for IT candidates. As a result the overall mortality of children in the US waiting for intestine graft is 3 fold higher compared to liver transplant candidates and reaches 251 deaths/1000 patient years on waiting list. Moreover post transplant survival rate for patients who are at home while waiting for transplantation is 15% higher than for those who undergo transplantation while in hospital [9], stressing again the benefit of early referral for transplant while the child is stable.

Beath et al., proposed in 2008 a set of referral criteria for children with intestinal failure (Table 1) to encourage practitioners to refer patients with early complications for transplant assessment and avoid late referrals with high mortality post listing [10].

The criteria recommend on early assessment in children with diseases and co-morbidities associated with poor prognosis such as massive intestinal resection, certain congenital diarrheas and early signs of IFALD or loss of vascular access. In a recent questionnaire based survey in IT centers it was found that approximately three fourth of the patients needing IT are referred late for pre-transplant assessment. This may be due to lack of knowledge and education of the referring hospitals or the fact that the criteria are considered by many as too general. The authors concluded that age based categories and formulation of a flow chart with specific decision points could be helpful [11].

Table 1. Refferal Criteria for children with IF

Children with massive intestine resection
Continuing prognostic or diagnostic uncertainty
Persistent hyperbilirubinemia (>6g/dl)
Children with severely diseased bowel and unacceptable morbidity
Microvillous inclusion disease or intestinal epithelial dysplasia
Thrombosis of 2 of 4 upper body central veins
Request of the patient or family

Those patients who are referred for pre-transplant assessment require a careful risk assessment to ascertain comparative survival of continuing non-transplantation therapy compared to predicted survival after transplantation. Prediction of who could achieve adequate intestinal adaptation especially in infants undergoing major intestinal resection is difficult [12]. Intestinal adaptation does not simply depend on the residual bowel length but also on etiology of IF, presence of associated complications from PN, quality of life (QOL) and expertise of the managing team. Thus, decision to list a patient is highly individualized and occasionally challenging.

IT remains the recommended therapy when all options to achieve intestinal adaptation have been exhausted. Current listing for IT is based on criterion proposed by The American Society of Transplantation in 2001 [13]:

1. Progressive intestinal failure associated liver disease with plasma bilirubin >3-6mg/dl and signs of portal hypertension, or synthetic liver dysfunction with coagulopathy
2. Recurrent life threatening episodes of sepsis resulting in multi-organ failure, metastatic infectious foci or acquisition of flora with limited antibiotic sensitivities
3. Loss of more than 50% of the standard central venous access sites
4. Small bowel length of <25 cm without an ileo-cecal valve
5. Congenital intractable mucosal disorder such as microvillous inclusion disease or tufting enteropathy, which usually leads to early death in infancy
6. Intestinal failure with high morbidity and poor quality of life

Intestinal failure-associated liver disease (IFALD) is the most common indication for IT in children. In a retrospective case series the incidence of IFALD leading to liver failure and death in infants with short bowel syndrome receiving PN has been reported to reach almost 25%[14, 15]. A study by

Pironi et al., where candidates for IT and non candidates were followed over 3 years in a prospective multicenter setting in Europe showed a survival advantage of IT for patients with liver failure due to PN. Three-year transplant free survival was 87% vs. 94% for candidates compared to non-candidates [16]. This supports the view of IT as a standard therapy for this subset of patients with IFALD. However, the report by Pironi et al., and data from our center question the validity of some of the listing criteria in the current era with improved outcome of children with intestinal failure. The 5 year survival of patients with disease specific criteria (bowel length and congenital diarrheas) or poor quality of life who remain on PN was better compared to IT recipients [17] and the positive predictive value and sensitivity of these criteria have dropped [18]. Careful and individualized assessment is needed in listings for these criteria to ensure improved long term patient survival.

Absolute and relative contraindications to IT are similar to other solid organ transplants and include life threatening and other non correctable illness not directly related to the digestive system, severe congenital or acquired immunological deficiencies, non resectable malignancies, multi system autoimmune diseases, profound neurologic disabilities and insufficient vascular patency to sustain central venous access for up to 6 months following transplantation [13].

Graft Types

There are three broad types of IT as shown in Figures 1-3: isolated intestine, combined liver-intestine and multivisceral (full or modified) [19].

Nomenclature in the modern era is derived from inclusion of specific organs. Intestine is the central core along with inclusion of liver and stomach defining the nomenclature.

Isolated IT is performed for patients with irreversible IF without any significant liver disease. It is indicated in patients with limited venous access, recurrent line infections, unmanageable fluid and electrolyte balance and reversible liver dysfunction with PN. Proximal donor jejunum is anastomosed to the recipient jejunum to restore intestinal continuity and an end ileostomy is created for surveillance. Vascular anastomosis comprises of donor superior mesenteric artery (SMA) to the recipient's SMA or native aorta. Venous drainage of the graft could be directed through the inferior vena cava or into the portal system of the recipient. Isolated IT is a preferred surgical option due to its shorter waiting time and the graft can be removed if necessary without compromising other organs. Isolated IT has been performed more often in adults (55%) compared to children (37%). Whereas combined liver-intestine is required more frequently for children (50%) compared to adults (21%) due to higher incidence of IFALD[20].

Combine liver-intestine was first described in 1990 by Grant et al., [21]. The Omaha group then described the current method of en-bloc dissection to include intestine, liver, duodenum and pancreas [22]. No donor portal dissection or biliary anastomosis is required in this method, an advantage in terms of surgical complexity and potential surgical complications. For composite grafts such as this and multivisceral grafts a donor aortic conduit is usually anastomosed to the recipient's infra-renal aorta. Proximal bowel is anastomosed end to end with recipient native bowel. The distal bowel is brought out as an end ileostomy or anastomosed end to end with recipient bowel, with creation of a proximal diverting loop ileostomy. Combined liver-intestine transplantation is indicated when IF is complicated by IFALD leading to significant portal hypertension, severe cholestasis, irreversible hepatocellular injury and porto-mesenteric venous thrombosis.

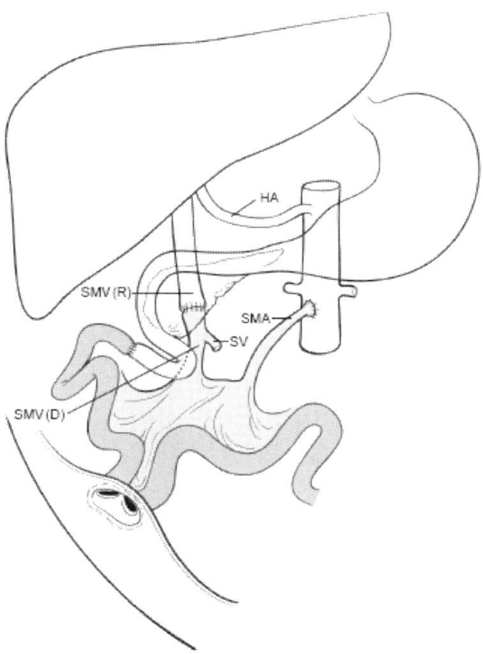

Figure 1. Isolated intestinal transplantation.

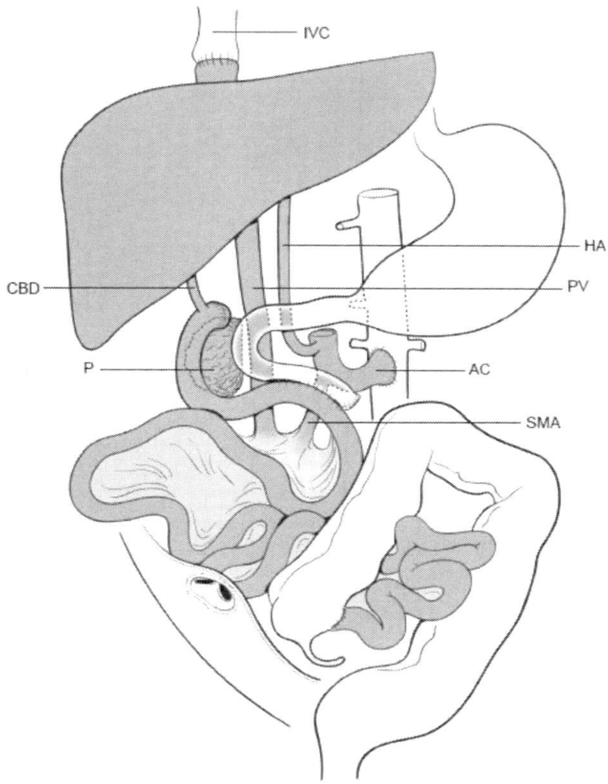

Figure 2. Combined liver-intestine transplantation.

Multivisceral transplantation (MVTx) comprises of other abdominal organs in addition to intestine and stomach such as duodenum, pancreas, spleen, kidney and possibly with liver (full multivisceral) or without liver (modified multivisceral). This en-bloc transplantation is done more commonly in adults (24%) compared to children (13%) [20]. Common indications in children for this procedure are severe motility disorders, locally aggressive but non-metastazing tumors, traumatic loss of abdominal viscera or extensive abdominal pathology that cannot be safely removed without an evisceration or reconstruction with multiple organs (e.g. children with multiple previous operations and severe portal hypertension). MVTx requires proximal gastrointestinal anastomosis between donor and recipient gastric fundus and a pyloroplasty as the stomach loses its vagal innervation. The remaining vascular anastomoses are similar to liver intestine allograft.

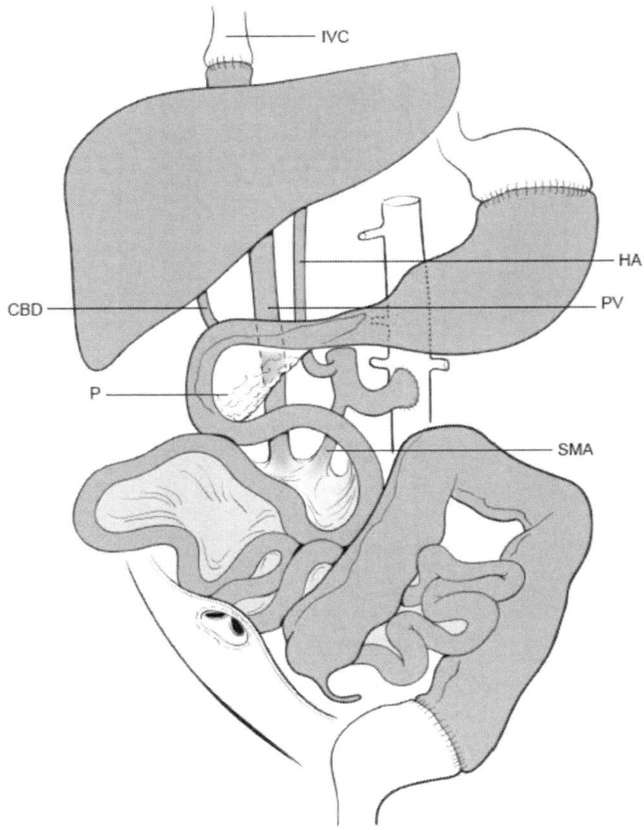

Figure 3. Multivisceral transplantation.

Inclusion of colon in the allograft of any of these 3 graft types had remained controversial until recently. Experimentally, colon has shown to slow intestinal transit time and improve absorption. Early studies suggested that it leads to increased bacterial load in the terminal ileum and translocation leading to increased rate of sepsis [23]. However, recent report from Kato and colleagues [24] has shown that inclusion of colon had no additional effect on morbidity or on graft survival and it improved QOL. Current opinion is to consider inclusion of colon where possible as it leads to enhanced water absorption, decreased motility and improved QOL [25].

In a very selected group of patients with IFALD who are close to achieving enteral autonomy and tolerates more than 50% of their calories via the enteral route, isolated liver transplantation could be considered as a rescue therapy. This option has to be reviewed and performed in experienced Intestinal rehabilitation centers with close links to IT team.

Post – Operative Management

Early Post-Operative Management

The early post transplantation course is affected by the graft type, patient status pre-transplant, donor characteristics, ischemia-reperfusion injury, graft acceptance and the degree of graft dysmotility. Patients require admission to the intensive care unit that is often relatively prolonged and warrants close monitoring. The early post-operative course requires maintenance of hemodynamic and fluid balance to ensure allograft perfusion without pulmonary fluid overload which could otherwise prolong the need for mechanical ventilation support. Routine monitoring in addition to routine ICU follow up includes Doppler ultrasound to assess the blood flow to the allograft and initiation of acute intestinal rejection surveillance.

Post-operative complications in this early phase usually relates to the surgery. Most common complications that could be encountered are chylous ascites, pleural effusion, peritonitis (non-perforating/perforating), stoma breakdown, hemorrhage, thrombosis of vascular anastomoses and bowel obstruction. Such surgical complications have been reported as low as 7.6% in a large center (n=500) secondary to significant improvements in the surgical technique [26].

Routine post-transplantation medical therapy includes prophylactic broad-spectrum antibiotics and antifungals, pneumocystis carinii prophylaxis with trimethoprim-sulfamethoxazole, CMV prophylaxis with ganciclovir depending on donor and recipient's status, proton pump inhibitor use and immunosuppressive therapy (discussed below).

Immunosuppression

Intestine graft rejection is more common, severe and difficult to prevent and treat compared to other solid organs because of the high immunogenicity of the gut. About 80% of the immune cells reside in the gut, which is repopulated with recipient immune cells within weeks of the transplant [27]. In addition, gut epithelium is not only involved in digestion and absorption but also plays a major role in intestine immunity and functions as a natural barrier for bacteria and foreign antigens. Epithelial cells and the gut mucosa take part in antigen presentation and allorecognition, innate and adaptive immunity interactions, and production of antibacterial peptides [28]. This heightened immunity with constant exposure to commensal flora, external microorganisms and foreign antigens in the presence of breached intestinal barrier (due to ischemia-reperfusion injury, recipient immune cells or defects such as impaired microbial control mechanisms) results in inflammation and tissue damage and lead to increased likelihood of acute rejection.

There are no randomized controlled trials for optimal immunosuppression strategies in IT recipients and current practices relies mostly on comparison with historical controls [29]. There are many variations in immunosuppressive protocols among transplant centers with similar outcomes. However there are significant similarities between transplant centers in some areas: need for allograft lymphocyte depletion with antibody induction for the recipient and a combination of calcineurin inhibitor (Tacrolimus) with high dose steroids based maintenance immunosuppression. Optimal immunosuppression forms the major determinant of the outcome as under-immunosuppression may lead to allograft rejection and over-immunosuppression has high risk for infections [30] and post transplant lympho-proliferative disorders (PTLD).

Most centers use induction therapy using lymphocyte-depleting agent such as rabbit antithymocyte globulin (Thymoglobulin), IL-2 blockers (Bailiximab) or alemtuzumab (Campath-1H) a monoclonal anti-CD52 antibody in addition to methylprednisone and tacrolimus at initial trough levels of 15-18 ng/ml. Using this type of protocols the acute rejection rate has been reported around 30%-50%[31-33]. Alemtuzumab has been associated with life threatening respiratory complications such as ARDS like illness, especially in young children. Thus, it should be used with caution in children less than 4 years[34]. Maintenance therapy with tacrolimus and low-dose corticosteroids, either alone or in combination with sirolimus (rapamycin) or Mycophenolate Mofetil (MMF), remains the most effective and reliable long-term regimen.

Many patients who require IT are sensitized due to history of multiple transfusions or re-transplantation. Predominant risk in these individuals is preformed or formation of donor-specific antibodies (DSA). Recent study has shown that a sensitized recipient with panel reactive antibodies (PRA) more than 20%, presence of DSA and positive cross-match was associated with poor outcome [35]. As a result complement dependent cytotoxic cross matching or virtual cross-match are performed by some centers before the transplant in order to minimize the risk of poor graft outcome due to antibody mediated rejection. In patients with a positive cross match screen additional administration of human immunoglobulin transfusion and plasmapheresis in combination with the routine induction protocol should be considered. In addition, the use of virtual cross match pre-transplant for allocation and reduction of immunologic risk in isolated intestine transplants was recently reported [36]. In this strategy organs were only offered to sensitized patients with DSA titers < 1:16. Rejection rate, graft and patient survival were comparable between sensitized and non-sensitized patients suggesting a role for cross match testing pre-transplant as a potential strategy to improve short-term outcome.

Surveillance for Allograft Rejection

Acute rejection (AR) is usually manifested in the form of diarrhea (increase in stoma output), but can also present as abdominal pain, fever, bloody diarrhea, change in stool habits and laboratory abnormalities such as anemia and hypoalbuminaemia [37]. Diarrhea however is a non-specific symptom and could be caused by a variety of etiologies that include graft rejection (acute and chronic), infections, immunosuppressive medications, dysmotility, lymphatic obstruction, neoplastic (PTLD/lymphoma) and fat malabsorption. Thus it warrants an urgent endoscopic evaluation to rule out AR and additional tests and evaluations based on the clinical suspicious for other potential etiologies.

AR occurs in up to half of the patients with IT and its early detection and prompt treatment remains a major determinant of patient and graft survival. Due to lack of a reliable clinical or tissue biomarker to differentiate between AR and infection, routine surveillance mucosal biopsies through the simple or loop ileostomy remains the mainstay for monitoring post IT. The optimal frequency of protocol ileoscopies for early detection of AR (i.e. before onset of clinical symptoms) is unknown but twice a week for the first month, followed by a gradual reduction in the frequency until stoma closure [37] is a common practice by many transplant centers. In situation of high suspicion of AR and normal ileal biopsy, an upper endoscopy with small bowel biopsies may have to be considered [20].

Although a few non-invasive markers for graft surveillance are described in the literature, the search continues for a reliable and sensitive marker that can conclusively differentiate between AR and infection and replace endoscopy. Unfortunately up to now a reliable marker has not been identified. Two markers, plasma citrulline level and stool calprotectin levels have generated major interest and are being studied extensively [38]. Citrulline is an amino acid that is primarily produced by enterocytes from conversion of glutamine [39]. Due to its enterocyte specific origin, it gained interest for monitoring enterocyte mass in IF patients and subsequently to monitor for enterocyte damage in patients with IT [40, 41]. Plasma citrulline has high intra-individual variability, influenced by kidney function and reaches a plateau around 90-120 days from transplantation, limiting its utility in the immediate post transplant phase [42]. Although low plasma citrulline level indicates mucosal damage, it does not differentiate well between rejection, infection, GVHD or PTLD [43, 44]. However citrulline may be used as a screening tool.for mucosal damage and levels less than 20 mmol/L are well correlated with the presence of acute rejection while levels of <10 mmol/L might indicate moderate – severe rejection [44]. In these cases low citrulline level should prompt an urgent endoscopy and mucosal biopsy for definite diagnosis. Calprotectin is a cytosolic protein from the s100 family of proteins. It is found in high concentration in the cytoplasm of neutrophils and can be detected in stool in the presence of active inflammation. Its use is inflammatory bowel disease and correlation to disease activity has been extensively studied. Sudan and colleagues were the first to report its utility in IT to detect AR. They found significant differences in median calprotectin levels between rejection and normal groups or viral enteritis groups on biopsies with a sensitivity of 83% and specificity of 77% [45]. Subsequent studies have not conclusively determined a generalizable cutoff value to confirm rejection, reported on significant interpatient variability and questioned the importance of calprotectin as a valuable screening method [46-48].

Nutrition

Principal objective of IT is establishing enteral autonomy with ability to consume an unrestricted age-appropriate diet and discontinuation of PN. There are no randomized controlled trials to define optimal nutritional rehabilitation and approach in the post transplant period. The simple aim is to commence enteral feeds as soon as possible. A survey conducted at the five largest transplant centers found that the average time to commence feeds was between 3-7 days, once the postoperative ileus had resolved [29].

Low volume feeds low in fat and osmolality are commenced in the early post transplant period to stimulate the digestive hormones and enzymes without provoking an osmotic diarrhea [49]. There are no consensus recommendations for the type of formula i.e. polymeric versus elemental; as a result it varies in different centers. Long chain triglycerides are avoided until 4-6 weeks post transplant period due to disruption of the lymphatic channels during the transplant surgery and diets with high medium chain triglycerides are recommended at this stage. Most children are commenced on continuous feeds for a few weeks and switched to bolus feeds as per tolerance.

Post transplant complications such as graft malfunction due to ischemia-reperfusion injury, acute rejection, infection, PTLD or anatomical factors (lymphatic disruption and denervation of bowel) can hamper tolerance of feeds and impact the pace of PN weaning. Food aversion is common in IT recipients and combined efforts of dieticians and oral therapist to promote oral intake of formula and solid food are important in the recovery and rehabilitation post transplant. Almost 45% of children are dependent on enteral tube feeds for complete or supplemental nutrition for the first 2 years after transplantation and 22% until 5 years [50]. As a result introduction of solid food in children is prolonged compared to that of adults and is restricted to low simple sugars, low fat and low osmolality to reduce risk of increased output.

Short Term and Long Term Complications

Acute Rejection

AR is the most important predictor of graft survival and death after IT [27]. Early detection and prompt treatment of AR will prevent progression to an uncontrolled rejection and are crucial for improved outcome. It is an immune mediated allograft injury involving both the cellular and humoral arms of immunity. Recent report suggest that IT recipients with nucleotide oligomerization domain-2 (NOD-2) polymorphism (a gene associated with Crohn's disease), show higher rate of rejection and graft failure [51] but this finding was not replicated by others. Polymorphism in NOD-2 predisposes to increased immunological response potentially due to inadequate microbial defense with epithelial damage, bacterial invasion and secondary inflammatory response. Pathologic criteria to define and grade AR were first published in 2003 by Wu et al., [52] followed by consensus criteria formulated at the 8th small bowel transplantation symposium and remains widely accepted [53]. AR is not isolated to the small bowel and can occur in any of the transplanted organs including liver, pancreas and colon.

Most AR episodes occurs in the first year post transplantation and more so during the first 90 days. Acute rejection previously occurred in up to 90% of IT patients. However with the advent of immunosuppression agents for induction therapy such as antithymocyte globulin, IL-2 blockers (Bailiximab) [32] or monoclonal anti-CD52 (alemtuzumab) [33] - rejection rate has reduced to 30% - 50%. Other factors that have shown to reduce AR are inclusion of a liver composite graft [54, 55], IT as a part of multivisceral transplantation [34], early detection due to surveillance ileoscopies and standardized histologic criteria to differentiate between rejection vs. infection [53].

Patients with AR can remain asymptomatic and diagnosed on surveillance ileoscopies or present with increased stoma output, diarrhea, fever, and intestinal obstruction or bleeding in severe exfoliative rejection [37]. In the absence of other definite non-invasive markers, histologic changes and grading of severity based on the accepted pathological criteria remains the cornerstone for diagnosis and management of AR. Endoscopic appearance of the mucosa could indicate severity i.e. no significant changes or mild erythema in mild rejection, erythema with focal erosion in moderate and extensive ulceration with separation of mucosa-submucosa with sloughing in severe exfoliative rejection. The severity of AR is determined by the presence and degree of characteristic histologic changes including crypt epithelial cell apoptosis and injury, villus damage with blunting, architectural distortion and edema with vascular congestion and inflammatory cell infiltrates. AR can be graded from 0 to 3 with 0 being no rejection to 3 being severe exfoliative rejection. Presence of some apoptosis (<6 apoptotic bodies/10 crypts) without fulfillment of the criteria for grade 1 is considered to be indeterminate and repeat biopsies are required to confirm the diagnosis. Exfoliative rejection carries high risk for graft loss and mortality in children with IT [56]. Early identification (before the patients become symptomatic or experiences higher grade of rejection on pathology) and treatment of AR ensures improved outcome.

Boluses of methylprednisolone with increase in trough level of Tacrolimus may suffice for mild-moderate rejection; moderate to severe rejection is usually treated with addition of antithymocye globulin (Thymoglobulin) to methylprednisolone. Emerging evidence support the use of Infliximab (Anti – Tumor Necrosis Factor α antagonist) as a salvage therapy in patients with late onset and potentially early onset steroid refractory and/or thymoglobulin resistant acute rejection [57, 58] and for chronic ulcerative ileitis.

Antibody mediated rejection (AMR) through preformed and de-novo donor specific antibodies (DSA) has emerged over the last decade as a leading cause for severe treatment refractory rejection, graft loss and chronic rejection [59, 60]. Presence of a liver graft has a protective effect and is associated with improved outcome. The diagnosis of antibody mediated rejection is not well established in IT and is based on the combination of severe acute rejection often refractory to conventional treatment, presence of DSA and occasionally histological vascular alterations. Unlike kidney transplantation C4d staining as a mean to diagnose AMR in IT is unreliable. It can be detected in both normal and rejecting grafts and its role in the diagnostic process is still unclear [61]. The treatment approach to AMR differs from the classical approach to T cell mediated AR and comprise of multimodal approach with elimination and inhibition of circulating Ab, suppression of B cell proliferation and complement inhibition [61].Response to Rituximab (Monoclonal antibody against B-lymphocyte CD20 receptor) and plasmapheresis with IVIg [62] has been observed, as these treatments reduce the concentration of circulating antibodies. Proteasome inhibitors like bortezomib has shown promise in these highly sensitized individuals with high levels of DSA and evidence of ongoing allograft injury [63]. Routine surveillance of DSA peri-operatively and post transplant is recommended to detect patient at risk for AMR.

Chronic Rejection

Chronic rejection (CR) is the most common but less well-defined cause of late onset graft dysfunction. CR is clinically suspected in the presence of diarrhea or increased stoma output that are unresponsive to escalation of anti-rejection therapy.

The hallmark of CR is obliterative endarteriopathy and intimal hyperplasia in the submucosal layers leading to progressive intestinal ischemia, fibrosis, stricture and graft loss [64]. Although endoscopic mucosal biopsies may demonstrate loss of villi, non-healing ulcer or fibrosis; a full thickness biopsy is needed to confirm the diagnosis. Patients with recurrent and severe AR or recipients of isolated IT are at a higher risk for CR [65]. In the absence of a definitive therapy resumption of PN and eventual re-transplantation is the only solution for patients with chronic rejection [37].

Infections

Infections remain a predominant cause of morbidity and mortality in children with IT. They are more susceptible to viral, bacterial and fungal infections due to profound immunosuppression, breach in the gut barrier due to AR or lympho-proliferative disorders and lack of natural immunity to viruses such as CMV or EBV due to transplants in infancy [66]. Infections can be categorized as: Allograft specific and systemic infections that affect the allograft.

Viral and bacterial enteritis may present with increased stoma output and is an ongoing challenge to differentiate from AR due to overlap in histological changes. Most commonly isolated organisms are Adenovirus, calicivirus, Clostridium difficile, and cytomegalovirus. Biopsy evaluation by a pathologist experienced in IT is warranted [67]. Histologic changes that may support the diagnosis of viral infection of the GI tract are thick mononuclear infiltrate adjacent to gut lumen, superficial apoptosis and most importantly abnormalities detected in the native bowel as well [37]. Use of immunohistochemistry and polymerase chain reaction may aid in the identification of virus on the biopsies. Patients with viral infection require careful fluid and electrolyte management until resolution of diarrhea.

Systemic bacterial infections are common in the first 6 months post IT. Being less than 18 years of age, inclusion of liver and pre transplant serum bilirubin level > 5mg/dl are risk factors for higher incidence of septicemia. Most common isolates are Enterococcus species, Enterobacter species, Klebsiella species, and coagulase-negative staphylococci [68]. Almost 91% of children experience at least 1 episode of infection after IT and MVTx with a median of 5 infectious episodes per child [34]. Although septicemia could be adequately treated with antibiotics, it remains one of the leading causes of death and accounts for 50% of deaths according to the intestinal transplant registry [9] and in many cases is associated with the occurrence of acute rejection.

The most important systemic viruses that affect children after IT are CMV, EBV and adenovirus. These are also among the leading causes of allograft loss and death because of their capacity to damage other vital organs such as liver, respiratory tract and central nervous system. The incidence of CMV infection in pediatric IT is close to 5% [69]. Highest risk of acquiring CMV infection is by placing a latently infected allograft in a CMV-naïve recipient. Routine screening of blood PCR along with variable combinations of intravenous ganciclovir, oral valganciclovir and cytogam (CMV immune globulin) for 3-12 months post transplantation remains mainstay for prophylaxis. Surveillance for EBV infection is important due to its predisposition for development of PTLD. Early detection with peripheral blood PCR has led to treatment before onset of disease or transition to PTLD. Reduction in immunosuppression and treatment with cytogam and ganciclovir can be used to treat EBV viraemia [70]. Adenovirus is seen more commonly with children especially in young infants and its incidence is as high as 20% [71]. Usual symptoms are fever, increase stoma output/diarrhea and respiratory tract involvement lasting for up to 2 weeks. Reduction in immunosuppression helps in viral clearance and treatment with cidofovir may be considered.

Other Complications

Post transplant Lympho-proliferative disorder (PTLD) is an EBV driven process due to proliferation of B-lymphocytes in the absence of EBV specific T-lymphocytes secondary to immunosuppressive therapy. As already mentioned improved surveillance of EBV and early treatment has led to significant reduction in the incidence of PTLD to current rate of 5 - 10% [27, 34, 69]. This rate is still higher compared to other solid organ transplants. Diarrhea, vomiting, fever and enlarged lymphoid mass in the usual sites (tonsils, adenoids, peripheral lymph nodes, lungs or native gut and mesentery) form the common symptom cluster of PTLD. PTLD can also lead to abnormal liver enzymes, white blood cell count, anemia and hypoalbuminemia. Viral load measurements through EBV PCR samples is an effective measure for monitoring while end organ biopsy is required to establish the diagnosis of PTLD. Although reduction in immunosuppression is effective in preventing EBV proliferation, it has to be balanced against the risk of AR. Reduction in immunosuppression is usually combined with Ganciclovir treatment in early stages of PTLD and high EBV viral load. Progressive PTLD warrants either treatment with Rituximab (Monoclonal antibody against B-lymphocyte CD20 receptor) that has shown up to 70% response [72, 73] or chemotherapy for resistant disease [72].

While graft versus host disease (GVHD) occurs in just about 5% of IT recipients, it is higher compared to other solid organ transplantation [34]. This could be explained by a rather large inoculum of donor lymphoid cells in the graft, especially for recipients of MVTx. It occurs more often in children compared to adults and recipients of MVTx compared to isolated intestinal or combined liver-IT [74]. The clinical presentation may include either erythematous maculopapular rash, deranged liver function in isolated IT, bone marrow suppression, dysphagia with esophageal involvement or blood-streaked diarrhea with involvement of the native colon. Mild disease responds to high dose steroids but progressive disease carries high mortality [34, 74].

Other comorbidities that are seen in children with IT are similar to other solid organ transplantation but their prevalence may be higher compared to other solid organ transplants due to higher dose and prolonged treatment periods of certain immunesuppressive medications. Drug induced progressive renal insufficiency is more common in IT compared to other solid organ transplantation and reaches an incidence of up to 21% in adult survivors after 5 years [75] leading to a fourfold increase in mortality. Risk factors for this high rate of renal insufficiency include high tacrolimus levels, low pre-operative GFR, admission to intensive care unit before transplantation, long term use of PN before and occasionally after the transplant and frequent episodes of significant fluid shifts and dehydration due to ongoing use of IV fluids and high stoma output [37]. Other side effects from combining steroids and tacrolimus are hypertension, hyperlipidemia and diabetes mellitus.

Outcome

More than 2600 IT have been performed worldwide (Intestinal transplant registry report 2011). There has been marked improvement in the short term graft and patient survival over the past decade with only modest improvements in the long term survival beyond 3 years after IT [67]. According to the last report of the international Intestinal Transplant Registry in 2011 the 1y patient survival for children who underwent IT transplant in 2006-2011 is 73% and the 5y survival is 55%. Better survival has been reported in high volume centers in United States and Europe compared to low volume centers with 3-year survival reaching 70% - 84% [37]. In the current era of immunosuppression, 1-, 3- and 5- year patient survival from Pittsburgh has been reported to be 95%, 84% and 77% respectively and graft survival of 88%, 74% and 58%[76]. Patient survival for isolated IT at 1, 3 and 5 years were 85%, 71.3% and 65% respectively and those with combined liver and intestine were 68.4%, 57% and 51.4% respectively. This shows improved survival for recipients of isolated IT in the first few years [77]. Use of a multivisceral (with or without liver) transplant, induction with daclizumab, patient at home prior to transplant, and age at transplant $\geq$ 1 year favorably influences patient survival [34]. Similar findings have been reported by the Intestinal Transplant registry where patients at home pre-transplant, patients at large volume centers and inclusion of liver graft had improved outcome while children younger than 1 year experienced reduced survival. Poor graft outcome is also associated with nonfunctional social support and these patients are at a greater risk for graft loss and death [78]. Remarkable improvement in the short-term outcome and modest long-term graft survival has led to increase in children requiring re-transplantation. The reported rate of re-transplantation is now reaching to 8% - 10% of all IT performed [26, 79]

The ultimate goal of IT is to achieve enteral autonomy and wean of PN. Most children surviving beyond 6 months are weaned off PN in 1-3 months with a median duration of 31 days. Weight gain is demonstrated in 6 months and vertical growth in 12 months but with limited catch up growth. Favorable predictors of weight gain and growth are shorter hospitalization, absence of rejection, low steroid usage and use of peptide-based formulas [80]. Almost half of the children who are successfully weaned off PN remain on tube feeding due to oral aversion that has developed over time pre-transplant. These children benefit from supplementation of extra calories to compensate for persistent fat malabsorption post transplant. Protein and carbohydrate absorption is usually normal [50, 81]. Micronutrient deficiencies (zinc, iron, and copper) are common post transplantation and need optimization [80].

Limited data exists on pediatric quality of life (QOL) after IT and in comparison to children on TPN. A recent study to compare QOL in adults on home TPN with patients post IT using HPN-QOL questionnaire demonstrated improvement in most aspects of QOL after IT [82]. However, children with median duration of follow up of 2.8 years post IT had significantly low Health-related QOL compared to normal children. Although Children with IT, did not self-report any difference in HR-QOL compared to normal children their school performance and psychosocial health along with parental report suggested otherwise. Preliminary studies show the contrasting QOL between adults and children; more studies in this area are warranted [83].

In summary, intestine transplantation should be the preferred treatment option for children with intestinal failure and life threatening complications related to TPN treatment. The overall short term outcome and survival of pediatric recipients of IT has significantly improved over the last 2 decades and most of the long term survivors achieve enteral autonomy and good social functioning and quality of life. On the other hand the long term patient and graft survival at 5 and 10 years post transplant has not changed significantly over the last decade. The unique immunologic features of the intestine and its role as a natural barrier with constant exposure to foreign antigens contribute to this guarded outcome. Development of strategies to prevent long term complications and improve long term outcome is the next challenge of IT.

References

[1] Starzl, TE; KHJ. Mass homotransplantation of abdominal organs in dogs. *Surg Forum.*, 1960(11), 28-30.

[2] Diliz-Perez, HS; McClure, J; Bedetti, C; Hong, HQ; de Santibanes, E; Shaw, BW; Jr., et al. Successful small bowel allotransplantation in dogs with cyclosporine and prednisone. *Transplantation.*, 1984, 37(2), 126-9.

[3] Pritchard, TJ; Kirkman, RL. Small bowel transplantation. *World Journal of Surgery.*, 1985, 9(6), 860-7.

[4] Diamond, IR; de Silva, N; Pencharz, PB; Kim, JH; Wales, PW. Neonatal short bowel syndrome outcomes after the establishment of the first Canadian multidisciplinary intestinal rehabilitation program: preliminary experience. *J Pediatr Surg.*, 2007, 42(5), 806-11. Epub 2007/05/16.

[5] Nucci, A; Burns, RC; Armah, T; Lowery, K; Yaworski, JA; Strohm, S; et al. Interdisciplinary management of pediatric intestinal failure: a 10-year review of rehabilitation and transplantation. *J Gastrointest Surg.*, 2008, 12(3), 429-35; discussion 35-6. Epub 2007/12/20.

[6] Torres, C; Sudan, D; Vanderhoof, J; Grant, W; Botha, J; Raynor, S; et al. Role of an intestinal rehabilitation program in the treatment of advanced intestinal failure. *J Pediatr Gastroenterol Nutr.*, 2007, 45(2), 204-12. Epub 2007/08/02.

[7] Goulet, O; Ruemmele, F; Lacaille, F; Colomb, V. Irreversible intestinal failure. *Journal of Pediatric Gastroenterology & Nutrition.*, 2004, 38(3), 250-69.

[8] Fecteau, A; Atkinson, P; Grant, D. Early referral is essential for successful pediatric small bowel transplantation: The Canadian experience. *Journal of Pediatric Surgery.*, 2001, 36(5), 681-4.

[9] Report of Intestine Transplant Registry: 25 years of Paediatric Follow-up. online: *Intestinal Transplant Associateion*, 2009.

[10] Beath, S; Pironi, L; Gabe, S; Horslen, S; Sudan, D; Mazeriegos, G; et al. Collaborative strategies to reduce mortality and morbidity in patients

with chronic intestinal failure including those who are referred for small bowel transplantation. *Transplantation.*, 2008, 85(10), 1378-84.

[11] Struijs, M-C; Sloots, CEJ; Tibboel, D; Ijzermans, JNM. The gap in referral criteria for pediatric intestinal transplantation. *Transplantation.*, 2012, 94(1), 92-8.

[12] Goulet, O; Sauvat, F. Short bowel syndrome and intestinal transplantation in children. Current Opinion in Clinical Nutrition & Metabolic Care. 2006, 9(3), 304-13.

[13] Kaufman, SS; Atkinson, JB; Bianchi, A; Goulet, OJ; Grant, D; Langnas, AN; et al. Indications for pediatric intestinal transplantation: a position paper of the American Society of Transplantation. *Pediatric Transplantation.*, 2001, 5(2), 80-7.

[14] Spencer, AU; Neaga, A; West, B; Safran, J; Brown, P; Btaiche, I; et al. Pediatric short bowel syndrome: redefining predictors of success. *Annals of Surgery.* , 2005, 242(3), 403-9, discussion 9-12.

[15] Wales, PW; de Silva, N; Kim, JH; Lecce, L; Sandhu, A; Moore, AM. Neonatal short bowel syndrome: a cohort study. *Journal of Pediatric Surgery.*, 2005, 40(5), 755-62.

[16] Pironi, L; Forbes, A; Joly, F; Colomb, V; Lyszkowska, M; Van Gossum, A; et al. Survival of patients identified as candidates for intestinal transplantation: a 3-year prospective follow-up. *Gastroenterology.*, 2008, 135(1), 61-71.

[17] Pironi, L; Joly, F; Forbes, A; Colomb, V; Lyszkowska, M; Baxter, J; et al. Long-term follow-up of patients on home parenteral nutrition in Europe: implications for intestinal transplantation. Gut., 2011, 60(1), 17-25.

[18] Karolina, M; Burghardt, PWW; Nicole, de Silva; David Grant, Yaron Avitzur. Relevance of Intestinal Transplant Criteria in the New Era of Specialised Care for Intestinal Failure. *XIII International Small Bowel Transplant Symposium - ISBTS 2013*, Oxford England2013.

[19] Abu-Elmagd, KM. The small bowel contained allografts: existing and proposed nomenclature. *American Journal of Transplantation.*, 2011, 11(1), 184-5.

[20] Abu-Elmagd, KM. Intestinal transplantation for short bowel syndrome and gastrointestinal failure: current consensus, rewarding outcomes, and practical guidelines. *Gastroenterology.*, 2006, 130(2 Suppl 1), S132-7.

[21] Grant, D; Wall, W; Mimeault, R; Zhong, R; Ghent, C; Garcia, B; et al. Successful small-bowel/liver transplantation. *Lancet.*, 1990, 335(8683), 181-4.

[22] Sudan, DL; Iyer, KR; Deroover, A; Chinnakotla, S; Fox, IJ; Jr. Shaw, BW; Jr., et al. A new technique for combined liver/small intestinal transplantation. *Transplantation.*, 2001, 72(11), 1846-8.

[23] Todo, S; Tzakis, A; Reyes, J; Abu-Elmagd, K; Furukawa, H; Nour, B; et al. Small intestinal transplantation in humans with or without the colon. *Transplantation.*, 1994, 57(6), 840-8.

[24] Kato, T; Selvaggi, G; Gaynor, JJ; Takahashi, H; Nishida, S; Moon, J; et al. Inclusion of donor colon and ileocecal valve in intestinal transplantation. *Transplantation.*, 2008, 86(2), 293-7.

[25] Matsumoto, CS; Kaufman, SS; Fishbein, TM. Inclusion of the colon in intestinal transplantation. *Current Opinion in Organ Transplantation.*, 2011, 16(3), 312-5.

[26] Abu-Elmagd, KM; Costa, G; Bond, GJ; Soltys, K; Sindhi, R; Wu, T; et al. Five hundred intestinal and multivisceral transplantations at a single center: major advances with new challenges. Annals of Surgery. 2009, 250(4), 567-81.

[27] Fishbein, TM. Intestinal transplantation. *New England Journal of Medicine.*, 2009, 361(10), 998-1008.

[28] Pirenne, J; Kawai, M. Intestinal transplantation: evolution in immunosuppression protocols. *Current Opinion in Organ Transplantation.*, 2009, 14(3), 250-5.

[29] Horslen, SP. Optimal management of the post-intestinal transplant patient. *Gastroenterology.*, 2006, 130(2 Suppl 1), S163-9.

[30] Garg, M; Jones, RM; Vaughan, RB; Testro, AG. Intestinal transplantation: current status and future directions. *Journal of Gastroenterology & Hepatology.*, 2011, 26(8), 1221-8.

[31] Abu-Elmagd, KM; Costa, G; Bond, GJ; Wu, T; Murase, N; Zeevi, A; et al. Evolution of the immunosuppressive strategies for the intestinal and multivisceral recipients with special reference to allograft immunity and achievement of partial tolerance. *Transplant International.*, 2009, 22(1), 96-109.

[32] Sudan, DL; Chinnakotla, S; Horslen, S; Iyer, K; Fox, I; Shaw, B; et al. Basiliximab decreases the incidence of acute rejection after ntestinal transplantation. *Transplantation Proceedings.*, 2002, 34(3), 940-1.

[33] Nishida, S; Levi, DM; Moon, JI; Madariaga, JR; Kato, T; Selvaggi, G; et al. Intestinal transplantation with alemtuzumab (Campath-1H) induction for adult patients. *Transplantation Proceedings.*, 2006, 38(6), 1747-9.

[34] Kato, T; Tzakis, AG; Selvaggi, G; Gaynor, JJ; David, AI; Bussotti, A; et al. Intestinal and multivisceral transplantation in children. *Annals of Surgery.*, 2006, 243(6), 756-64, discussion 64-6.

[35] Farmer, DG; Venick, RS; Colangelo, J; Esmailian, Y; Yersiz, H; Duffy, JP; et al. Pretransplant predictors of survival after intestinal transplantation: analysis of a single-center experience of more than 100 transplants. *Transplantation.*, 2010, 90(12), 1574-80.

[36] Hawksworth, JS; R-BS, Island, E; Girlanda, R; Guerra, JF; Valdiconza, C; Kishiyama, K; Christensen, KD; Kozlowski, S; Kaufman, S; Little, C; Shetty, K; Laurin, J; Satoskar, R; Kallakury, B; Fishbein, TM; Matsumoto, CS. Successful isolated intestinal transplantation in sensitized recipients with the use of virtual crossmatching. *American Journal of Transplantation.*, 2012 Dec(12), Suppl 4, S33-42. Epub 2012 Sep 4.

[37] Avitzur, Y; Grant, D. Intestine transplantation in children: update 2010. *Pediatric Clinics of North America.*, 2010, 57(2), 415-31, table of contents.

[38] Mercer, DF. Hot topics in postsmall bowel transplantation: noninvasive graft monitoring including stool calprotectin and plasma citrulline. *Current Opinion in Organ Transplantation.*, 2011, 16(3), 316-22.

[39] Curis, E; Crenn, P; Cynober, L. Citrulline and the gut. *Current Opinion in Clinical Nutrition & Metabolic Care.*, 2007, 10(5), 620-6.

[40] Pappas, PA; Saudubray, JM; Tzakis, AG; Rabier, D; Carreno, MR; Gomez-Marin, O; et al. Serum citrulline and rejection in small bowel transplantation: a preliminary report. *Transplantation.*, 2001, 72(7), 1212-6.

[41] Crenn, P; Coudray-Lucas, C; Thuillier, F; Cynober, L; Messing, B. Postabsorptive plasma citrulline concentration is a marker of absorptive enterocyte mass and intestinal failure in humans. *Gastroenterology.*, 2000, 119(6), 1496-505.

[42] Gondolesi, GE; Kaufman, SS; Sansaricq, C; Magid, MS; Raymond, K; Iledan, LP; et al. Defining normal plasma citrulline in intestinal transplant recipients. *American Journal of Transplantation.*, 2004, 4(3), 414-8.

[43] Gondolesi, G; Ghirardo, S; Raymond, K; Hoppenhauer, L; Surillo, D; Rumbo, C; et al. The value of plasma citrulline to predict mucosal injury in intestinal allografts. *American Journal of Transplantation.*, 2006, 6(11), 2786-90.

[44] Hibi, T NS; Garcia, J; Tryphonopoulos, P; Tekin, A; Selvaggi, G; Weppler, D; Levi, DM; Ruiz, P; Tzakis, AG. Citrulline level is a potent indicator of acute rejection in the long term following pediatric intestinal/multivisceral transplantation. *American Journal of Transplantation.*, 2012, 12(December), Suppl 4, S27-32. Epub 2012 Jul 19.

[45] Sudan, D; Vargas, L; Sun, Y; Bok, L; Dijkstra, G; Langnas, A; Calprotectin: a novel noninvasive marker for intestinal allograft monitoring. *Annals of Surgery.*, 2007, 246(2), 311-5.

[46] Akpinar, E; Vargas, J; Kato, T; Smith, L; Hernandez, E; Selvaggi, G; et al. Fecal calprotectin level measurements in small bowel allograft monitoring: a pilot study. *Transplantation.*, 2008, 85(9), 1281-6.

[47] Cagnola, H; Scaravonati, R; Cabanne, A; Bianchi, C; Gruz, F; Errea, A; et al. Evaluation of calprotectin level in intestinal content as an early marker for graft rejection. *Transplantation Proceedings.*, 2010, 42(1), 57-61.

[48] Mercer, DF; Vargas, L; Sun, Y; Moreno, AMA; Grant, WJ; Botha, JF; et al. Stool calprotectin monitoring after small intestine transplantation. *Transplantation.*, 2011, 91(10), 1166-71.

[49] Gupte, GL; Beath, SV. Update on intestinal rehabilitation after intestinal transplantation. *Current Opinion in Organ Transplantation.*, 2009, 14(3), 267-73.

[50] Lacaille, F; Vass, N; Sauvat, F; Canioni, D; Colomb, V; Talbotec, C; et al. Long-term outcome, growth and digestive function in children 2 to 18 years after intestinal transplantation. *Gut.*, 2008, 57(4), 455-61.

[51] Fishbein, T; Novitskiy, G; Mishra, L; Matsumoto, C; Kaufman, S; Goyal, S; et al. NOD2-expressing bone marrow-derived cells appear to regulate epithelial innate immunity of the transplanted human small intestine. *Gut.*, 2008, 57(3), 323-30.

[52] Wu, T; Abu-Elmagd, K; Bond, G; Nalesnik, MA; Randhawa, P; Demetris, AJ. A schema for histologic grading of small intestine allograft acute rejection. *Transplantation.*, 2003, 75(8), 1241-8.

[53] Ruiz, P; Bagni, A; Brown, R; Cortina, G; Harpaz, N; Magid, MS; et al. Histological criteria for the identification of acute cellular rejection in human small bowel allografts: results of the pathology workshop at the VIII International Small Bowel Transplant Symposium. *Transplantation Proceedings.*, 2004, 36(2), 335-7.

[54] Middleton, SJ; Jamieson, NV. The current status of small bowel transplantation in the UK and internationally. *Gut.*, 2005, 54(11), 1650-7.

[55] Jugie, M; Canioni, D; Le Bihan, C; Sarnacki, S; Revillon, Y; Jan, D; et al. Study of the impact of liver transplantation on the outcome of intestinal grafts in children. *Transplantation.*, 2006, 81(7), 992-7.

[56] Ishii, T; Mazariegos, GV; Bueno, J; Ohwada, S; Reyes, J. Exfoliative rejection after intestinal transplantation in children. *Pediatric Transplantation.*, 2003, 7(3), 185-91.

[57] Gerlach, UA; Koch, M; Muller, HP; Veltzke-Schlieker, W; Neuhaus, P; Pascher, A. Tumor necrosis factor alpha inhibitors as immunomodulatory antirejection agents after intestinal transplantation. American Journal of *Transplantation.*, 2011, 11(5), 1041-50.

[58] De Greef, E; Avitzur, Y; Grant, D; De-Angelis, M; Ng V; Jones, N; et al. Infliximab as salvage therapy in paediatric intestinal transplant with steroid- and thymoglobulin-resistant late acute rejection. *Journal of Pediatric Gastroenterology & Nutrition.*, 2012, 54(4), 565-7.

[59] Abu-Elmagd, KM; Costa, WG; Lunz, G; Martin, J; Koritsky, L; DA, Murase, N; Irish, W; Zeevi, A. Preformed and de novo donor specific antibodies in visceral transplantation: long-term outcome with special reference to the liver. *American Journal of Transplantation.*, 2012, Nov(12), 3047-60. Epub 2012 Sep 4.

[60] Association Between Donor-Specific Antibodies and Acute Rejection and Resolution in Small Bowel and Multivisceral Transplantation. *Transplantation September.*, 2011, 92(6), 709-15.

[61] Antibody-mediated rejection after intestinal transplantation. *Current Opinion in Organ Transplantation June.*, 2012, 17(3), 250-7.

[62] Ruiz, P; Carreno, M; Weppler, D; Gomez, C; Island, E; Selvaggi, G; et al. Immediate antibody-mediated (hyperacute) rejection in small-bowel transplantation and relationship to cross-match status and donor-specific C4d-binding antibodies: case report. *Transplantation Proceedings.*, 2010, 42(1), 95-9.

[63] Gerlach, UA; Schoenemann, C; Lachmann, N; Koch, M; Pascher, A. Salvage therapy for refractory rejection and persistence of donor-specific antibodies after intestinal transplantation using the proteasome inhibitor bortezomib. *Transplant International.*, 2011, 24(5), e43-5.

[64] Noguchi, Si; S-i, Reyes, J; Mazariegos, GV; Parizhskaya, M; Jaffe, R; Pediatric intestinal transplantation: the resected allograft. *Pediatric & Developmental Pathology.*, 2002, 5(1), 3-21.

[65] Parizhskaya, M; Redondo, C; Demetris, A; Jaffe, R; Reyes, J; Ruppert, K; et al. Chronic rejection of small bowel grafts: pediatric and adult study of risk factors and morphologic progression. *Pediatric & Developmental Pathology.*, 2003, 6(3), 240-50.

[66] Sigurdsson, L; Reyes, J; Kocoshis, SA; Mazariegos, G; Abu-Elmagd, K; Green, M. Bacteremia after intestinal transplantation in children correlates temporally with rejection or gastrointestinal lymphoproliferative disease. *Transplantation.*, 2000, 70(2), 302-5.

[67] Pironi, L; Staun, M; Van Gossum, A. Intestinal transplantation. *New England Journal of Medicine.*, 2009, 361(24), 2388-9, author reply 9.

[68] Akhter, K; Timpone, J; Matsumoto, C; Fishbein, T; Kaufman, S; Kumar, P. Six-month incidence of bloodstream infections in intestinal transplant patients. *Transplant Infectious Disease.*, 2012, 14(3), 242-7.

[69] Bond, GJ; Mazariegos, GV; Sindhi, R; Abu-Elmagd, KM; Reyes, J. Evolutionary experience with immunosuppression in pediatric intestinal transplantation. *Journal of Pediatric Surgery.*, 2005, 40(1), 274-9, discussion 9-80.

[70] Humar, A; Hebert, D; Davies, HD; Humar, A; Stephens, D; O'Doherty, B; et al. A randomized trial of ganciclovir versus ganciclovir plus immune globulin for prophylaxis against Epstein-Barr virus related posttransplant lymphoproliferative disorder. *Transplantation.*, 2006, 81(6), 856-61.

[71] McLaughlin, GE; Delis, S; Kashimawo, L; Cantwell, GP; Mittal, N; Cirocco, RE; et al. Adenovirus infection in pediatric liver and intestinal transplant recipients: utility of DNA detection by PCR. *American Journal of Transplantation.*, 2003, 3(2), 224-8.

[72] Elstrom, RL; Andreadis, C; Aqui, NA; Ahya, VN; Bloom, RD; Brozena, SC; et al. Treatment of PTLD with rituximab or chemotherapy. *American Journal of Transplantation.*, 2006, 6(3), 569-76.

[73] Codeluppi, M; Cocchi, S; Guaraldi, G; Di Benedetto, F; Bagni, A; Pecorari, M; et al. Rituximab as treatment of posttransplant lymphoproliferative disorder in patients who underwent small bowel/multivisceral transplantation: report of three cases. *Transplantation Proceedings.*, 2005, 37(6), 2634-5.

[74] Mazariegos, GV; Abu-Elmagd, K; Jaffe, R; Bond, G; Sindhi, R; Martin, L; et al. Graft versus host disease in intestinal transplantation. American *Journal of Transplantation.*, 2004, 4(9), 1459-65.

[75] Ojo, AO; Held, PJ; Port, FK; Wolfe, RA; Leichtman, AB; Young, EW; et al. Chronic renal failure after transplantation of a nonrenal organ. *New England Journal of Medicine.*, 2003, 349(10), 931-40.
[76] Mazariegos, GV; Squires, RH; Sindhi, RK. Current perspectives on pediatric intestinal transplantation. *Current Gastroenterology Reports.*, 2009, 11(3), 226-33.
[77] KM, DCMFGAGRK. Age-Based Disparity in Outcomes of Intestinal Transplants in Pediatric Patients. *American Journal of Transplantation*, 2012(12), S43–S8.
[78] Long-Term Survival, Nutritional Autonomy, and Quality of Life After Intestinal and Multivisceral Transplantation. *Annals of Surgery September.*, 2012, 256(3), 494-508.
[79] Pediatric Intestinal Retransplantation: Techniques, Management, and Outcomes. *Transplantation December.*, 2008, 86(12), 1777-82.
[80] Venick, RS; Wozniak, LJ; Colangelo, J; Beckwith, P; Reyen, L; Esmailian, YA; et al. Long-term nutrition and predictors of growth and weight gain following pediatric intestinal transplantation. *Transplantation.*, 2011, 92(9), 1058-62.
[81] Intestinal absorption rate in children after small intestinal transplantation. *Am J Clin Nutr.*, 2013, 6, 6.
[82] Assessment of quality of life on home parenteral nutrition and after intestinal transplantation using treatment-specific questionnaires. *Am J Transplant.*, 2012, 12(Suppl 4), S60-6. doi: 10.1111/j.600-6143.2012.04244.x. Epub 2012 Sep 7.
[83] Ngo, KD; Farmer, DG; McDiarmid, SV; Artavia, K; Ament, ME; Vargas, J; et al. Pediatric health-related quality of life after intestinal transplantation. *Pediatric Transplantation.*, 2011, 15(8), 849-54.

In: Short Bowel Syndrome in Children
Editor: Igor Sukhotnik
ISBN: 978-1-62948-518-8

Chapter XI

Tissue Engineering and Regenerative Medicine Research Perspectives for Intestinal Failure

Amulya K. Saxena, M.D.[*]
Department of Pediatric and Adolescent Surgery,
Head of Unit for Experimental Fetal Surgery and Tissue Engineering,
Medical University of Graz, Graz, Austria

Abstract

The recent advances in tissue engineering are of special interest to the pediatric surgical community. Tissue engineering is a multidisciplinary field, combining the principles of engineering and biological sciences with the aim of regenerating diseased or damaged tissues and organs. Generally, in tissue engineering, patient's own cells are isolated and then proliferated *in-vitro* and combined with a supportive scaffold. A scaffold material primarily provides a supportive structure onto which cells can attach and be confined and is generally categorized as natural or synthetic. In intestine, the *Hybrid Construct* concept utilizes

[*] Corresponding author: Prof. Dr. Amulya K. Saxena, Email: amulya.saxena@medunigraz.at.

specially fabricated scaffolds for a specific cell type for attachment to create cell-specific constructs, and layers the constructs of different cell types in the order that these are located in natural tissue. Tissue engineering presents a potential solution to the shortage of organs for organ transplant in the pediatric community and is therefore predicted to create a strong impact on the future of pediatric surgery.

1. Introduction

Current options for the replacement of loss tissue include transplantation, surgical reconstruction, medical devices and replacement therapies, all strategies that are associated with a range of problems and complications [1]. Transplantation is of particular concern, since there is an acute shortage of organ donors, especially in the pediatric age group [2]. In the event that suitable donors are identified, organ rejection and toxic effects of life-long immunosuppressants present further limitations in the treatment [3, 4, 5]. Tissue engineering and regenerative medicine has been proposed as an alternative strategy for the treatment of tissue loss. Tissue engineering is a multidisciplinary field, combining the principles of engineering and biological sciences with the aim of regenerating diseased or damaged tissues and organs (Figure 1).

Generally, in tissue engineering, patient's own cells are isolated and then proliferated *in-vitro* and combined with a supportive scaffold. The resulting cell/scaffold construct is then cultured *in-vitro* within a bioreactor, a device which mimics normal physiological conditions by providing physical stimulation to encourage cell growth and tissue-specific organization (Figure 2). Finally, the construct may be transplanted to the defect site [6,7,8].

Within the basic framework, there exist numerous alternative strategies of tissue engineering. The principle differences among those approaches lie in the choice of cell source and scaffold material. In some approaches, allogeneic cells may be applied instead of autologous cells, with the advantage of availability of larger cell numbers and the ability to create an *off-the-shelf* tissue engineering product, however, with the disadvantage of potential immunological rejection and disease [9]. With autologous cells, immune rejection would not be an issue; however, potentially, available cells may be limited in numbers, the required time for culturing (in order to achieve the required the critical number for seeding density) may be too long, or the patient's own cells may be unsuitable due to disease.

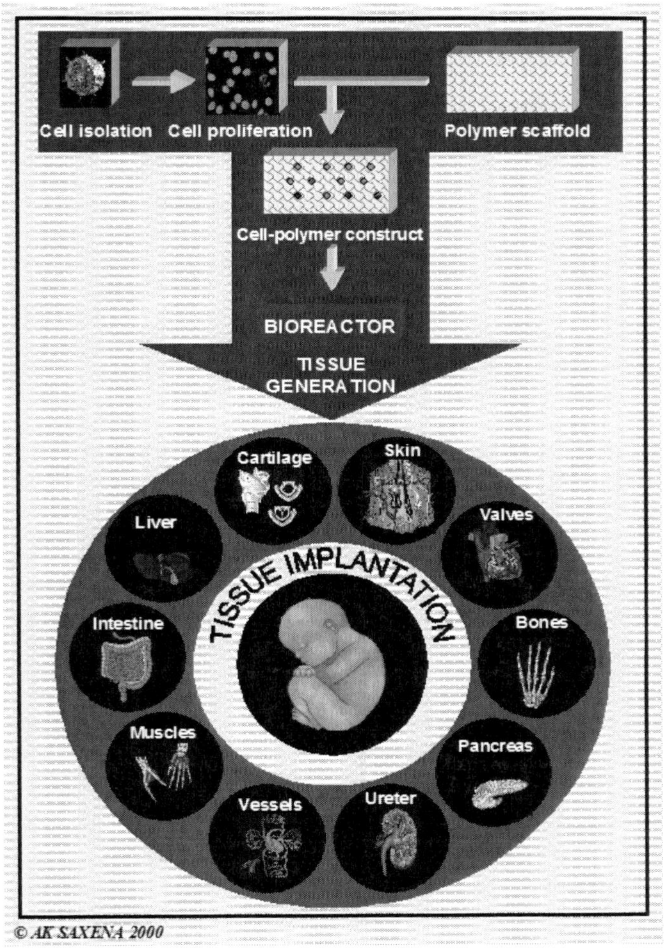

Figure 1. Overview of the principles of tissue engineering and regenerative medicine.

For both approaches, the proliferation of cells to obtain sufficient cell densities for therapeutic applications is a common difficulty. Mature cells derived from biopsies often are reluctant to proliferate in-vitro, and may be subject to de-differentiation. Therefore, the use of stem cells has gained increasing popularity in tissue engineering research.

Stem cells benefit principally from a high proliferative capacity, allowing for the isolation of large numbers of cells from relatively small biopsy samples.

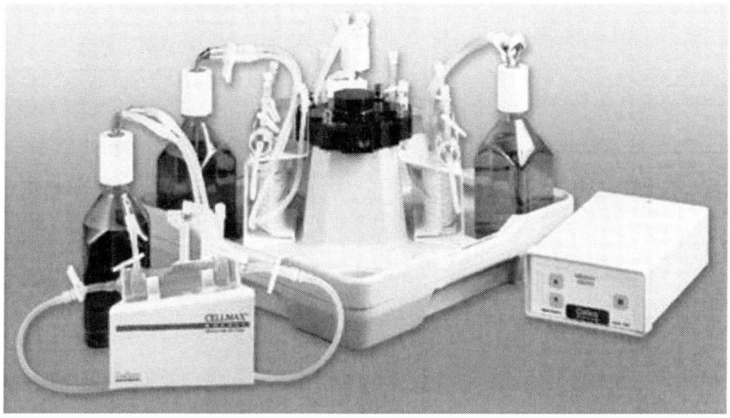

Figure 2. Bioreactor system used for in-vitro dynamic tissue generation. Nutrients are delivered to the cultivation chamber using a pump. Constant circulation facilitates better integration of the construct components. (Image: Cellmax Hollow Fiber Cell Culture System- with permission Spectrum Europe BV, Breda, The Netherlands).

In recent times, mesenchymal stem cells (MSCs) have received a great deal of attention [10]. MSCs can be isolated from a wide variety of tissue types and have the ability to differentiate into mesenchymal lineages [11]. Traditionally, MSCs have been isolated from bone marrow; however, MSCs derived from alternative sources, such as adipose tissue, are more easily isolated and may result in a more effective expansion of cell population [12]. The plasticity of MSCs is not as good as that of embryonic stem cells (ESCs); however, the use of ESCs is complicated by ethical issues and uncertainty as to whether such cells can be consistently differentiated into a target cell type [13]. Other promising sources of stem cells are those of the umbilical cord and amnion. Such cells are believed to show greater plasticity in comparison to adult MSCs, yet avoid the ethical dilemmas associated with the use of ESCs [14,15].

The second factor of importance in tissue engineering is the selection of an appropriate scaffold. A scaffold material primarily provides a supportive structure onto which cells can attach and be confined (Figure 3). The employment of a scaffold material has a number of benefits over simple injection of cells into a defect site:

- Firstly, the scaffold material localizes the cells to the defect site and restricts cell loss [16].

- A scaffold material also provides mechanical support to the defect site, which is of particular importance in the regeneration of structural tissues.
- As of such, it is desirable that a scaffold material mimics the biomechanical properties of the native tissue with regards to, for example, tensile strength and elasticity [17].
- A scaffold material must also be biocompatible, not illicit an inflammatory reaction, and have a rate of biodegradation which matches the rate of new tissue formation.

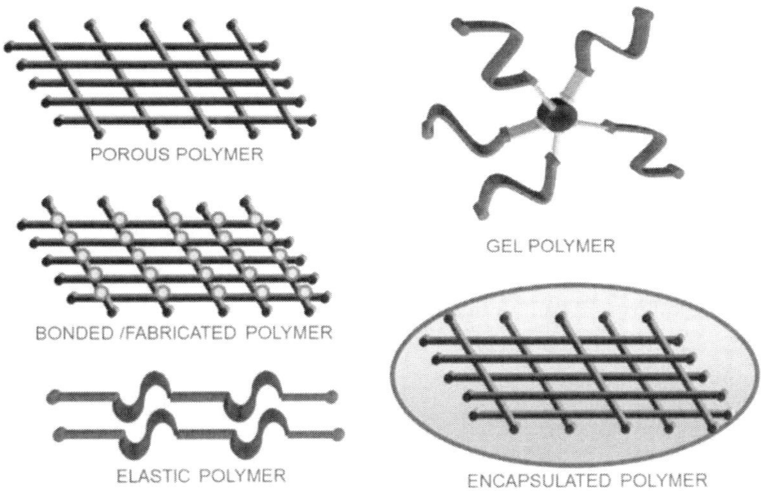

Figure 3. Schematic overview of basic scaffold types used for tissue engineering depending on the area of application and type of tissue that has to be generated.

Scaffold materials are generally categorized as natural or synthetic. Natural materials include decellularized tissue, in which cellular and nuclear materials have been removed from a donor tissue leaving only the extracellular matrix, or processed extracellular matrix scaffolds in which a naturally occurring protein, such as collagen, is purified and fabricated into a porous 3D material suitable for the infiltration of cells [18, 19].

Synthetic materials include polymers, bioceramics and bioglass. Polymers, in particular, benefit from the increased flexibility in design of novel materials with specific degradation rates, biomechanics, and their ability to be combined with other polymers to modify the resulting properties [20]. Scaffold materials can also be combined with a variety of growth factors to promote tissue growth and regulate tissue formation [21]. Finally, numerous studies have also demonstrated that tissues can be formed without a supportive scaffold, thus avoiding the issue of foreign body reactions. Examples of such approaches include self-assembling blood vessels and cell sheet technology for the formation of cardiac tissue [22, 23].

As with any new therapeutic technique, there are certain ethical issues that need to be addressed. The ethical issues that dominate debate on tissue engineering tend to be focused on the use of cells, in particular embryonic stem cells [23]. Other issues of importance include the use of adequate animal models in the experimental phase and weighing the risks and benefits for the patient during the clinical phase [24]. It has also been suggested that the inherent complexity of the tissue engineering processes could present a challenge to the informed consent process [25,26].

The true potential of tissue engineering is only beginning to be realized as research starts to be transferred into the clinical setting. The tissue engineering approach has already been applied in patients for the treatment of vessels, bladder, bronchus, cartilage and bone [27,28,29,30,31]. It is hoped that the next decade will see a significant increase in such clinical trials in which the actual benefit of tissue engineering can be assessed. This review will encompass current research in tissue engineering related to the main systems of the body with special emphasis on state-of-the-art research and clinical trials.

2. Tissue Engineering in Pediatric Surgery

The broadest spectrum of patients and pathologies are managed by the pediatric surgical community. Pediatric surgery involves surgical procedures on the fetus through the adolescent age groups, and is performed on a large range of organ systems. Congenital defects in particular, present a challenging task for the pediatric surgeon [32,33]. The significant loss of functional tissue mass, in such cases, is often beyond the natural regenerative processes of the body. Current techniques for the treatment of disorders, such as short bowel syndrome, suffer from many well-known limitations. Critically, the shortage of donor tissues for transplantation is a large problem for the pediatric age groups. In particular, waiting times for organ donation in the 0-5 year age range are considerably longer than other age groups [2]. For these reasons, the emergence of tissue engineering technology is of particular interest to the pediatric surgical community.

3. Short Bowel Syndrome and Tissue Engineering

Tissue engineering for Short Bowel Syndrome presents challenges that spill beyond the "simple" generation of the tubular small intestine. Patients with Short Bowel Syndrome have varying degree of liver manifestation; hence the advances in hepatic tissue engineering are also cover in this chapter. The small intestine not only a structural organ but also a function organ with an extreme complex nerve innervation. The advances with regards to nerve regeneration have also been elaborated to better explain the complexity of the challenges in intestinal tissue engineering.

4. Small Intestinal Tissue Engineering

Tissue engineering of the intestine is beset by problems caused by the complex anatomy and numerous functions of the intestine. This is unfortunate considering the potential benefit of a tissue engineered intestine for pediatric surgery. Intestinal tissue loss results from surgical resection in the treatment of a variety of diseases and disorders, including necrotising enterocolitis, volvulus and gastroschisis which may result in short bowel syndrome. The current option of treatment is transplantation, which despite significant improvements in the last decade, has a 5 year survival rate of just 75% in the best centers [34].

Synthetic conduits are largely unsuitable for rectifying small bowel syndrome as it is not just a case of loss of intestinal length, but more a case of loss of functional tissue capable of nutritional uptake. The goal of a tissue engineered intestinal tissue, therefore, is the provision of a functional tubular intestinal replacement containing a mucosa and associated vasculature capable of nutrient absorption and a muscular layer for participation in peristalsis. Early attempts at intestinal tissue engineering involved the seeding onto scaffolds of epithelial organoid units [35]. Organoid units can be produced by partial disruption of intestinal tissue through mechanical and enzymatic means. The units benefit from retaining the epithelial-mesenchymal cell-cell interaction which may be critical for cell survival and intestinal development. Organoid units attached to PGA scaffolds were implanted into the omentum of rats. The implanted organoid units showed proliferation and regeneration of larger complex structures with columnar epithelium, goblet cells, Paneth's cells and a crypt-villus-like morphology. Evidence that tissue engineered intestine can restore functionality has also been reported in the small animal model. Tissue engineered colon and small intestine were implanted in the rodent model, resulting in improved physiological and biochemical function and regaining of weight [36, 37].

More recently, the application of organoid units in the large animal model has shown promising results [38]. A 10 cm jejunum section was resected from swine piglets and closed by anastomosis. The resected tissue was processed for the isolation of organoid units, which were seeded onto nonwoven, PGA tubular scaffolds coated with 5% poly-L-lactic acid (PLLA) and type I collagen. The scaffolds were 3.5 cm in length with a diameter of 84 mm. The constructs were then implanted into the omentum or mesentery for a period of 7 weeks. Tissue engineered intestine was shown to possess a morphology similar to that of native tissue, with comparable villi length and crypt depth. The intestinal epithelial cells of tissue engineered intestine contained enterocytes, goblet cells and enteroendocrine cells. Both native and engineered tissue showed smooth-muscle muscularis and the presence of ganglion cells.

A concern over the use of organoid units is the poor survival rate after periods of prolonged *in vitro* culture. An alternative cell source which can be expanded *in vitro* to provide sufficient cells for therapeutic use may still be required. One such cell type which has shown promise is the amniotic stem cell which has shown to have a protective effect in animal models of necrotising enterocolitis [39]. In general, further studies are warranted for the development of intestinal tissue engineering. In particular, the determination of suitable cell sources and strategies for differentiation into the various cell types which constitute the intestinal wall. Furthermore, future tissue engineered constructs will have to undergo a series of biochemical and physiological tests to prove functionality.

Challenges in the tissue engineering of the small intestine have been underestimated with regards to the complexity of this simple hollow organ. As reported in experimental studies in intestinal tissue engineering, only simple scaffolds have been utilized in the regeneration of intestinal tissue. The complexity of the multiple cells involved in the engineering of hollow organs such as intestine, led our group to present the concept of "*Hybrid Construct*" for hollow organ tissue engineering in 2010 [40]. The *Hybrid Construct* concept utilizes specially fabricated scaffolds for a specific cell type for attachment to create cell-specific constructs, and layers the constructs of different cell types in the order that these are located in natural tissue (Figure 4).

In such as way cell-specific construct sheets can be amalgamated with each other over a stent to custom tailor the engineered hollow organ. Various surgical techniques for proper suturing of scaffolds to form hollow organs have been investigated for hollow organ tissue engineering [40]. Our group has investigated different scaffolds (natural, synthetic and composites) with regards to the formations of *Hybrid Construct* to determine the optimal scaffold for hollow organ tissue engineering [41]. For, gastrointestinal hollow organ tissue engineering, our group has employed the omentum as an *in-situ* bioreactor for hollow organ construct implantation and have demonstrated using micro computed tomography, the imaging of these constructs in the rodent model [42].

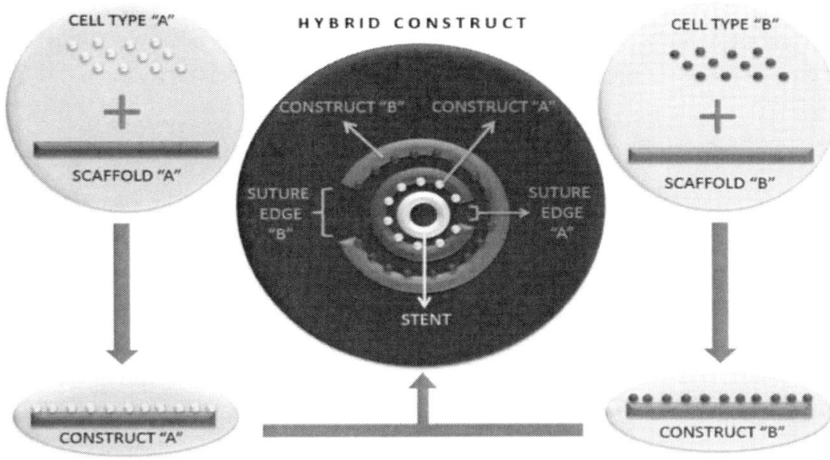

Figure 4. Schematic view of the *Hybrid Construct* concept applied for tissue engineering of hollow tubular organs.

Advances with the development of smooth muscle *Hybrid Construct* layer for esophagus can be translated for the tissue engineering of the small intestine. Scanning electron microscopic studies were performed by our group to evaluate the transformation of constructs to tissue and to better understand smooth muscle tissue generation under *in-vitro* conditions [43]. For proper functioning of smooth muscle tissue within the hollow organ in question (in this case the intestine) will depend on the rhythmic contraction of the cells to generate movement of the tissue.

Evaluation of our scaffolds by scanning electron microscopic investigation demonstrated the disorganized structure of the scaffold which led to disorganized tissue formation. The importance of scaffold micro-structure was evaluated and specially designed that were unidirectional were fabricated from porcine tendon collagen which were then employed to generate strands of smooth muscle tissue with proper orientation [44].

The challenges which confront intestinal tissue engineering are the questions of cell sourcing, designing and fabrication of scaffolds for *hybrid constructs* and in the better understanding of the complex micro-structure of the intestinal tissue.

Generation of large segments of hollow organs using *hybrid constructs* is being investigated by our group in the ovine model using multiple cell-specific scaffolds to engineer tissues of substantial size that could be utilized in future for transposition(Figure 5 and 6). The results emerging from these investigations are being evaluation carefully to improve the quality of engineered tissue in the large animal model set-up.

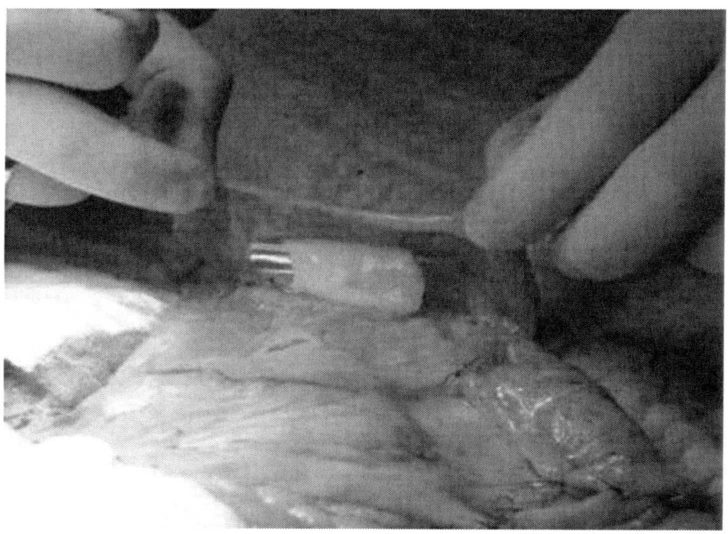

Figure 5. Operative view of a construct being wrapped into the omentum for in-situ tissue engineering in an ovine model.

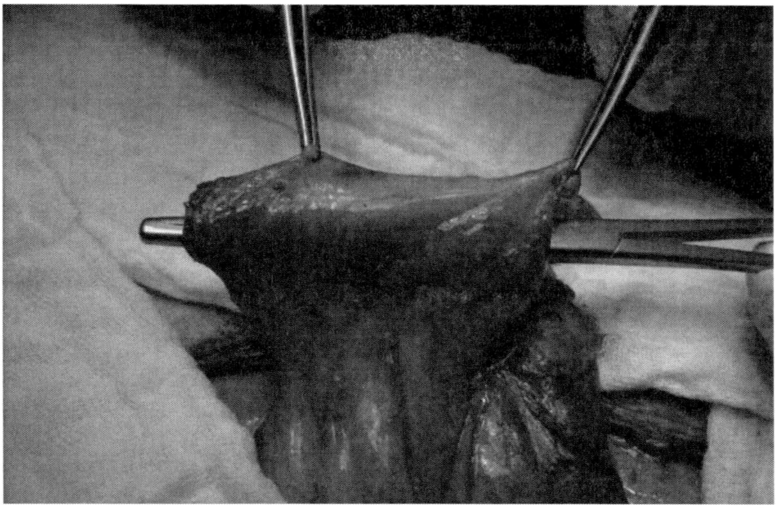

Figure 6. Operative view of a vascularized hollow organ construct and tissue generation in an ovine model 12 weeks after implantation which can be employed for transposition.

5. Liver Tissue Engineering

Short bowel syndrome is associated with varying degrees of associated liver pathology. End-stage liver disease in children requires liver transplantation; however, donor shortage and issues of immunosuppression present major limitations. Previous studies have demonstrated that transplantation of hepatocytes with a mass, equivalent to 10% of the patient's liver, may be sufficient for the correction of many enzyme deficiencies [45]. Currently, there exist two main approaches for hepatocyte transplantation [46]. The first involves transplantation of hepatocytes into the spleen or portal vein, resulting in engraftment of the cells within the host liver. Despite encouraging results, such a technique presents a risk of portal vein thrombosis and pulmonary embolism [47]. The second approach involves transplantation of hepatocytes beneath the kidney capsule or in other heterotopic sites [48].

To optimize the delivery and survival of hepatocytes, research has investigated the application of a tissue engineered hepatic transplantation. In this approach, a matrix is used as a carrier for the hepatocytes, allowing for the formation of a three-dimensional neo-tissue. Such a matrix could be coated with extracellular matrix (ECM) molecules or bound with growth factors to enhance engraftment and vascularization [49, 50]. Another benefit of localizing cells is that hepatocytes are dependent on cell-cell contact and ECM compositions for the maintenance of liver-specific function [51]. Combination of hepatocytes with a scaffold material also allows the cells to be cultured within an *in vitro* bioreactor. The application of bioreactors for hepatocyte culture has an important role in future developments of hepatic tissue engineering. Bioreactors are able to mimic the *in vivo* conditions present in the liver lobule including perfusion and oxygen tension, and studies have shown that culturing hepatocytes under flow conditions results in significant increases in cell number and enhanced cell function [49, 52].

The potential drawbacks with the use of synthetic scaffolds for hepatic tissue engineering are inflammation and fibrosis. By applying cell-sheet technology, a uniform and continuous sheet of hepatic tissue can be created without the requirement for a supportive scaffold. Furthermore, the resulting sheets can be layered *in vivo* to produce a three-dimensional construct, providing increased opportunities for cell-cell contact [53]. In such a study, primary hepatocytes were isolated from mouse livers and cells with high viabilities, determined by trypan blue dye exclusion test, were selected. The high-viability hepatocytes were plated onto temperature-responsive poly(*N*-isopropylacrylamide) (PIPAAm) polymers, cultured until confluent and subsequently harvested by temperature reduction. Ten days before implantation in the mouse, a subcutaneous space was prepared by implantation of a basic fibroblast growth factor (bFGF)-releasing mesh for the creation of a highly vascularized platform. The mesh was later removed and the hepatocyte cell-sheet was transplanted onto the vascularized platform. Additional sheets were then implanted directly on top of the first sheet to create a bilayer or 4-layer hepatic tissue.

The implanted cell-sheets showed prolonged survival of at least 235 days. In comparison to cells transplanted in the conventional method via the portal vein, subcutaneously implanted hepatocyte cell-sheets showed enhanced function and improved survival rates. The hepatocyte cell-sheets were shown to maintain phenotype and were capable of metabolizing circulating chemical compounds. In addition, the engineered tissue was shown to proliferate and grow in response to regenerative stimulus from resection of two-thirds of the liver. The strategy of implantation into a pre-vascularized subcutaneous site has notable advantages. Subcutaneous implantation is minimally invasive and allows for multiple transplantations with relative easy, whilst the vascularized platform increases engraftment and persistence of viability [53].

Such technology holds great promise for future therapies in the treatment of liver diseases. In the present status, engineered liver tissue cannot replace whole organ transplantation, as the current engineered tissue is unable to generate biliary connections to the intestine. Furthermore, the problem of hepatocyte proliferation remains unresolved. The use of stem cells differentiated towards a hepatic lineage may offer an alternative to primary hepatocytes. A variety of stem cells including, bone marrow derived MSCs, hematopoietic stem cells and fetal liver progenitor cells have shown to be effective in the treatment of liver disease [54, 55, 56]. The development of such strategies will be the focus of future research.

6. Advances in Nerve Tissue Engineering

The small intestine has an extremely complex intrinsic and extrinsic nerve innervation and any attempts to engineer small intestine without integrating the innervation will be unsuccessful. Hence, understanding of the advances in nerve tissue engineering will be of paramount importance if success of small intestinal tissue engineering has to be applicable at the level of the clinics. The regeneration of injured nerves is a complex challenge, yet potential improvement to a patient's quality of life would be vast. Spinal cord injuries in the pediatric population are relatively rare, with an average annual incident of 1.9 per 10^6 children below the age of 18; however, the consequences can be devastating [57]. Traumatic injury to the peripheral nervous system can also result in severe disability and most commonly occurs through obstetric and iatrogenic lesions, traffic accidents and lacerations [58]. In addition to traumatic injuries, numerous congenital disorders result from abnormalities of the peripheral and enteric nervous system, such as Hirschsprung's disease, in which regeneration of the nervous tissue would be of great advantage [59].

Regeneration of a severed spinal cord is complicated by the degenerative processes which follow severance. After cutting of the spinal cord, a massive release of lyosomal hydrolases causes autolysis of the cord stump, resulting in cavitation [60]. If the gap is too wide, or filled with scar tissue, spontaneous re-innervations will not occur. Therefore, to aid re-innervation across the defect site, researchers have developed biomaterial conduits with topographical and chemotactic signals, aimed at guiding nerve growth [61].

Tissue engineering has gained increasing popularity in the research of nerve repair. In particular for the peripheral nerve injuries, tissue engineering is seen as the most important field of future research, ahead of new surgical and medical techniques, and the use of xenografts [62]. In the tissue engineering approach, regenerative cells may be seeded within the biomaterial conduit. Numerous cell types have been proposed for use in nerve regeneration of both the peripheral and central nervous systems, including Schwann cells, Olfactory ensheathing cells, neural stem cells and MSCs [63, 64, 65, 66].

Some of the most promising studies involve the use conduits filled with Schwann cells, due to the cell's ability to remyelinate axons and secrete neurotrophic factors which promote nerve survival and axonal regeneration [67, 68]. In such a study, Schwann cells were seeded onto collagen gel sheets, which were subsequently rolled to form a conduit [69]. Neuronal cells were seen to migrate into the center of the conduit, through the inter-layered space. Significantly, the inward migration of the neuronal cells did not occur in conduits without Schwann cells.

Other studies have attempted to enhance the function of Schwann cells through transfection. For example, Schwann cells transfected with glial cell line-derived neurotrophic factor (GDNF), were shown to increase survival of motor neurons and improve nerve regeneration in a rat sciatic nerve defect [63].

In addition to glial cells, tissue engineered conduits containing neuronal cells have also been developed, which are of particular interest for the repair of longer nerve defects [70]. To produce a neuronal construct bridged by longitudinally orientated axons, recent research has utilized the ability of axons to grow in length in response to a continuous mechanical tension. Neurons from the dorsal root ganglia were isolated from fetal rats and cultured in media supplemented with mitotic inhibitors to limit the proliferation of glial cells. The explants were then plated as two populations at either end of two overlapping collagen-coated Aclar membranes. Axonal outgrowth across the membranes integrated the two explants. Next, the membranes were gradually separated over a period of 7 days. The mechanical tension induced stretch-growth of the axons, resulting in axonal tracts of 12-13 mm in length. The cell culture was embedded in a collagen-based matrix and inserted into a PGA Neurotube™. The constructs were then implanted into a 1 cm defect in the rat sciatic nerve and sutured to the epineurium and left for between 6 and 16 weeks. The neurons were shown to survive implantation and the construct architecture of longitudinally aligned axonal tracts was preserved. The maintenance of a neuronal phenotype was also verified through expression of neuronal cytoskeletal protein NF-200. The transplanted nerve processes were observed to penetrate at least 5 mm into the host nerve. Most importantly, host axons were identified growing into the proximal ends of the construct resulting in intimate contact between host axons and transplanted neurites. A similar approach was also applied to spinal cord injuries in the rodent model [71]. In this study, mechanically elongated dorsal root ganglia neurons, embedded in a collagen hydrogel, were used to bridge a 10 mm defect. The implanted cells were shown to survive for 4 weeks and implanted axons were observed extending into host spinal cord tissue.

The major concern with nerve tissue engineering is safety. It is important that no adverse reactions are produced by implanted biomaterials or cells. The threat of tumor-genesis from the use of stem cells is of particular concern; however, whilst the risk is very much real, it has also been suggested that this can be reduced through a rigorous selection for cells displaying regulated growth and cell cycle control, and a correct pattern of gene expression [72]. In 2009, Geron *Inc.* were granted permission to enter clinical trials with a human ESC therapy for the treatment of thoracic-level spinal cord injury [73]. The product approved for trials, contains human ESC-derived oligodendrocyte progenitor cells. Oligodendrocytes are able to remyelinate axons and also to produce neurotrophic factors which enhance the survival and function of neurones [74]. The results of this trial will be eagerly awaited by the tissue engineering community.

Summary and Future Perspectives

A great deal of effort and financing has been invested over the last two decades into tissue engineering as a solution for tissue and organ loss. At this point in time, data from early clinical trials are beginning to emerge and the results are promising. The success of tissue engineering depends largely on the complexity of the target organ in terms of anatomy and function. It is therefore of little surprise that the tissue types targeted by early tissue engineering clinical trials are relatively simple in form and function. In comparison, tissue engineering of the more complex tissues, consisting of multiple cell types and tissue components, are still some way from clinical trials. A major challenge in tissue engineering is the improved proliferation of cells in order to produce sufficient cell numbers. One potential solution is the use of stem cells, which have relatively high proliferative capacities; however, delivering consistent differentiation towards a target cell type remains a challenge.

The recent advances in tissue engineering are of special interest to the pediatric surgical community. Clinical trials in the pediatric population have already commenced; however, it should also be noted that the efficacy and safety of the tissue engineering approach has not yet been fully understood and such questions remain to be answered. Tissue engineering presents a potential solution to the shortage of organs for organ transplant in the pediatric community and is therefore predicted to create a strong impact on the future of pediatric surgery.

References

[1] Saxena, AK. Tissue engineering: Present concepts and strategies. *J Indian Assoc Pediatr Surg*, 2005, 10, 14-9.

[2] Eurotransplant International Foundation Annual Report 2008. Eds. Oosterlee A, Rahmel A. *Eurotransplant International Foundation, Leiden, The Netherlands.*, ISBN-13, 978-90-71658-28-0.

[3] Harada, KM; Mandia-Sampaio, EL; de Sandes-Freitas, TV; Felipe, CR; Park, SI; Pinheiro-Machado, PG; Garcia, R; Tedesco-Silva, H; Jr, Medina-Pestana, JO. Risk factors associated with graft loss and patient survival after kidney transplantation. *Transplant Proc.*, 2009, 41(9), 3667-70.

[4] Reding, R. Long-term complications of immunosuppression in pediatric liver recipients. *Acta Gastroenterol Belg.*, 2005, 68(4), 453-6.

[5] Magee, JC; Krishnan, SM; Benfield, MR; Hsu, DT; Shneider, BL. Pediatric transplantation in the United States, 1997-2006. *Am J Transplant.*, 2008, 8(4 Pt 2), 935-45.

[6] Langer, R; Vacanti, JP; Vacanti, CA; Atala, A; Freed, LE; Vunjak-Novakovic, G. Tissue engineering: biomedical applications. *Tissue Eng.*, 1995, 1(2), 151-61.

[7] Sistino, JJ. Bioreactors for tissue engineering--a new role for perfusionists? *J Extra Corpor Technol.*, 2003, 35(3), 200-2.

[8] Takeda, T; Vacanti, JP. Hepatocyte transplantation in the dalmatian dog model of hyperuricosuria. *Tissue Eng.*,1995, 1(4), 355-60.

[9] Lukish, JR; Eichelberger, MR; Newman, KD; Pao, M; Nobuhara, K; Keating, M; Golonka, N; Pratsch, G; Misra, V; Valladares, E; Johnson, P; Gilbert, JC; Powell, DM; Hartman, GE. The use of a bioactive skin

substitute decreases length of stay for pediatric burn patients. *J Pediatr Surg.*, 2001, 36(8), 1118-21.

[10] Caplan, AI. Mesenchymal stem cells. *J Orthop Res.*, 1991, 9(5), 641-50.

[11] Maniatopoulos, C; Sodek, J; Melcher, AH. Bone formation in vitro by stromal cells obtained from bone marrow of young adult rats. *Cell Tissue Res.*, 1988, 254(2), 317-30.

[12] Nakagami, H; Morishita, R; Maeda, K; Kikuchi, Y; Ogihara, T; Kaneda, Y. Adipose tissue-derived stromal cells as a novel option for regenerative cell therapy. *J Atheroscler Thromb.*, 2006, 13(2), 77-81.

[13] Vacanti, CA. History of tissue engineering and a glimpse into its future. *Tissue Eng.*, 2006, 12(5), 1137-42.

[14] Chen, MY; Lie, PC; Li, ZL; Wei, X. Endothelial differentiation of Wharton's jelly-derived mesenchymal stem cells in comparison with bone marrow-derived mesenchymal stem cells. *Exp Hematol.*, 2009, 37(5), 629-40.

[15] Roubelakis, MG; Pappa, KI; Bitsika, V; Zagoura, D; Vlahou, A; Papadaki, HA; Antsaklis, A; Anagnou, NP. Molecular and proteomic characterization of human mesenchymal stem cells derived from amniotic fluid: comparison to bone marrow mesenchymal stem cells. *Stem Cells Dev.*, 2007, 16(6), 931-52.

[16] Thorrez, L; Shansky, J; Wang, L; Fast, L; VandenDriessche, T; Chuah, M; Mooney, D; Vandenburgh, H. Growth, differentiation, transplantation and survival of human skeletal myofibers on biodegradable scaffolds. *Biomaterials.*, 2008, 29(1), 75-84.

[17] Kim, BS; Mooney, DJ. Scaffolds for engineering smooth muscle under cyclic mechanical strain conditions. *J Biomech Eng.*, 2000, 122(3), 210-5.

[18] Teebken, OE; Bader, A; Steinhoff, G; Haverich, A. Tissue engineering of vascular grafts: human cell seeding of decellularised porcine matrix. *Eur J Vasc Endovasc Surg.*, 2000, 19(4), 381-6.

[19] Kemp, PD; Cavallaro, JF; Hastings, DN. Effects of carbodiimide crosslinking and load environment on the remodeling of collagen scaffolds. *Tissue Eng.*, 1995, 1(1), 71-9.

[20] Freed, LE; Vunjak-Novakovic, G; Biron, RJ; Eagles, DB; Lesnoy, DC; Barlow, SK; Langer, R. Biodegradable polymer scaffolds for tissue engineering. *Biotechnology* (N Y)., 1994, 12(7), 689-93.

[21] Murphy, WL; Peters, MC; Kohn; DH; Mooney, DJ. Sustained release of vascular endothelial growth factor from mineralized poly(lactide-co-

glycolide) scaffolds for tissue engineering. *Biomaterials.*, 2000, 21(24), 2521-7.

[22] Kelm, JM; Lorber, V; Snedeker, JG; Schmidt, D; Broggini-Tenzer, A; Weisstanner, M; Odermatt, B; Mol, A; Zünd, G; Hoerstrup, SP. A novel concept for scaffold-free vessel tissue engineering: self-assembly of microtissue building blocks. *J Biotechnol.*, 2010, 148(1), 46-55. Epub 2010 Mar 17.

[23] Shimizu, T; Yamato, M; Kikuchi, A; Okano, T. Cell sheet engineering for myocardial tissue reconstruction. *Biomaterials.*, 2003, 24(13), 2309-16.

[24] de Vries, RB; Oerlemans, A, Trommelmans L, Dierickx K, Gordijn B. Ethical aspects of tissue engineering: a review. *Tissue Eng Part B Rev.*, 2008, 14(4), 367-75.

[25] Oerlemans, AJ; Rodrigues, CH; Verkerk, MA; van den Berg, PP; Dekkers, WJ. Ethical aspects of soft tissue engineering for congenital birth defects in children--what do experts in the field say? *Tissue Eng Part B Rev.*, 2010, 16(4), 397-403.

[26] Trommelmans, L; Selling, J; Dierickx, K. Ethical reflections on clinical trials with human tissue engineered products. *J Med Ethics.*, 2008, 34(9), e1.

[27] Hibino, N; Imai, Y; Shin-oka, T; Aoki, M; Watanabe, M; Kosaka, Y; Matsumura, G; Konuma, T; Toyama, S; Murata, A; Naito, Y; Miyake, T. First successful clinical application of tissue engineered blood vessel. *Kyobu Geka.*, 2002, 55(5), 368-73.

[28] Atala, A; Bauer, SB; Soker, S; Yoo, JJ; Retik, AB. Tissue-engineered autologous bladders for patients needing cystoplasty. *Lancet.*, 2006, 367(9518), 1241-6.

[29] Macchiarini, P; Jungebluth, P; Go, T; Asnaghi, MA; Rees, LE; Cogan, TA; Dodson, A; Martorell, J; Bellini, S; Parnigotto, PP; Dickinson, SC; Hollander, AP; Mantero, S; Conconi, MT; Birchall, MA. Clinical transplantation of a tissue-engineered airway. *Lancet.*, 2008, 372(9655), 2023-30.

[30] Adachi, N; Ochi, M; Deie, M; Ito, Y; Izuta, Y. Lateral compartment osteoarthritis of the knee after meniscectomy treated by the transplantation of tissue-engineered cartilage and osteochondral plug. *Arthroscopy.*, 2006, 22(1), 107-12.

[31] Meijer, GJ; de Bruijn, JD; Koole, R; van Blitterswijk, CA. Cell based bone tissue engineering in jaw defects. *Biomaterials.*, 2008, 29(21), 3053-61.

[32] Saxena, AK. Tissue engineering and regenerative medicine research perspectives for pediatric surgery. *Pediatr Surg Int.*, 2010, 26, 557-573.

[33] Saxena, AK. Congenital anomalies of soft tissues: birth defects depending on tissue engineering solutions and present advances in regenerative medicine. *Tissue Eng Part B.*, 2010, 16, 455-466.

[34] Avitzur, Y; Grant, D. Intestine transplantation in children: update 2010. *Pediatr Clin North Am.*, 2010, 57(2), 415-31.

[35] Choi, RS; Vacanti, JP. Preliminary studies of tissue-engineered intestine using isolated epithelial organoid units on tubular synthetic biodegradable scaffolds. *Transplant Proc.*, 1997, 29(1-2), 848-51.

[36] Grikscheit, TC; Ogilvie, JB; Ochoa, ER; Alsberg, E; Mooney, D; Vacanti, JP. Tissue-engineered colon exhibits function in vivo. *Surgery.*, 2002, 132(2), 200-4.

[37] Grikscheit, TC; Siddique, A; Ochoa, ER; Srinivasan, A; Alsberg, E; Hodin, RA; Vacanti, JP. Tissue-engineered small intestine improves recovery after massive small bowel resection. *Ann Surg.*, 2004, 240(5), 748-54.

[38] Sala, FG; Kunisaki, SM; Ochoa, ER; Vacanti, J; Grikscheit, TC. Tissue-engineered small intestine and stomach form from autologous tissue in a preclinical large animal model. *J Surg Res.*, 2009, 156(2), 205-12.

[39] Zani, A; Cananzi, M; Eaton, S; Pierro, A; De Coppi, P. Stem cells as a potential treatment of necrotizing enterocolitis. *J Pediatr Surg.*, 2009, 44(3), 659-60.

[40] Soltysiak, P; Höllwarth, ME; Saxena, AK. Comparisson of suture techniques in the formation of collagen scaffold tubes for composite tubular organ tissue engineering. *Biomed Mater Eng*, 2010, 20, 1-11.

[41] Saxena, AK; Damen, WF; van Kuppevelt, TH; Weijnen, R; Ainoedhofer, H; Höllwarth, ME. Comparison of collagen scaffold tubes for possible esophagus organ tissue engineering applications: In-situ omental implantation study in an ovine model. *Eur Surg.*, 2010, 42, 309-313

[42] Soltysiak, P; Saxena, AK. Micro-computed tomography for implantation site imaging during in situ oesophagus tissue engineering in a live small animal model. *J Tissue Eng Regen Med.*, 2009, 3, 573-576.

[43] Kofler, K; Leitinger, G; Kristler, M; Saxena, AK. Smooth muscle tissue engineering for hybrid tubular organs: scanning electron microscopic investigations of cell interactions with collagen scaffolds. *J Tissue Eng Regen Med.*, 2009, 3, 321-324.

[44] Saxena, AK; Kofler, K; Ainödhofer, H; Höllwarth, ME. Esophagus tissue engineering: hybrid approach with esophageal epithelium and unidirectional smooth muscle tissue component generation in vitro. *J Gastrointest Surg.*, 2009, 13, 1037-1043.

[45] Asonuma, K; Gilbert, JC; Stein, JE; Takeda, T; Vacanti, JP. Quantitation of transplanted hepatic mass necessary to cure the Gunn rat model of hyperbilirubinemia. *J Pediatr Surg.*, 1992, 27(3), 298-301.

[46] Fiegel, HC; Kneser, U; Kluth, D; Metzger, R; Till, H; Rolle, U. Development of hepatic tissue engineering. *Pediatr Surg Int.*, 2009, 25(8), 667-73.

[47] Nieto, JA; Escandón, J; Betancor, C; Ramos, J; Cantón, T; Cuervas-Mons, V. Evidence that temporary complete occlusion of splenic vessels prevents massive embolization and sudden death associated with intrasplenic hepatocellular transplantation. *Transplantation.*, 1989, 47(3), 449-50.

[48] Arkadopoulos, N; Papalois, A; Pataryas, TH, Golematis, B; Papadimitriou, J. Experimental transplantation of hepatocytes in cases of toxic acute liver failure. An allograft model. *Transpl Int.*, 1994, 7 Suppl 1, S171-4.

[49] Fiegel, HC; Havers, J; Kneser, U; Smith, MK; Moeller, T; Kluth, D; Mooney, DJ; Rogiers, X; Kaufmann, PM. Influence of flow conditions and matrix coatings on growth and differentiation of three-dimensionally cultured rat hepatocytes. *Tissue Eng.*, 2004, 10(1-2), 165-74.

[50] Lee, H; Cusick, RA; Browne, F; Ho Kim, T; Ma, PX; Utsunomiya, H; Langer, R; Vacanti, JP. Local delivery of basic fibroblast growth factor increases both angiogenesis and engraftment of hepatocytes in tissue-engineered polymer devices. *Transplantation.*, 2002, 73(10), 1589-93.

[51] Ambrosino, G; Basso, SM; Varotto, S; Zardi, E; Picardi, A; D'Amico, DF. Isolated hepatocytes versus hepatocyte spheroids: in vitro culture of rat hepatocytes. *Cell Transplant.*, 2005, 14(6), 397-401.

[52] Allen, JW; Khetani, SR; Bhatia, SN. In vitro zonation and toxicity in a hepatocyte bioreactor. *Toxicol Sci.*, 2005, 84(1), 110-9.

[53] Ohashi, K; Yokoyama, T; Yamato, M; Kuge, H; Kanehiro, H; Tsutsumi, M; Amanuma, T; Iwata, H; Yang, J; Okano, T; Nakajima, Y. Engineering functional two- and three-dimensional liver systems in vivo using hepatic tissue sheets. *Nat Med.*, 2007, 13(7), 880-5.

[54] Kharaziha, P; Hellström, PM; Noorinayer, B; Farzaneh, F; Aghajani, K; Jafari, F; Telkabadi, M; Atashi, A; Honardoost, M; Zali, MR; Soleimani, M. Improvement of liver function in liver cirrhosis patients after

autologous mesenchymal stem cell injection: a phase I-II clinical trial. *Eur J Gastroenterol Hepatol.*, 2009, 21(10), 1199-205.

[55] Salama, H; Zekri, AR; Zern, M; Bahnassy, A; Loutfy, S; Shalaby, S; Vigen, C; Burke, W; Mostafa, M; Medhat, E; Alfi, O; Huttinger, E. Autologous hematopoietic stem cell transplantation in 48 patients with end-stage chronic liver diseases. *Cell Transplant.*, 2010.

[56] Khan, AA; Shaik, MV; Parveen, N; Rajendraprasad, A; Aleem, MA; Habeeb, MA; Srinivas, G; Raj, TA; Tiwari, SK; Kumaresan, K; Venkateswarlu, J; Pande, G; Habibullah, CM. Human fetal liver-derived stem cell transplantation as supportive modality in the management of end-stage decompensated liver cirrhosis. *Cell Transplant.*, 2010, 19(4), 409-18.

[57] Puisto, V; Kääriäinen, S; Impinen, A; Parkkila, T; Vartiainen, E; Jalanko, T; Pakarinen, MP; Helenius, I. Incidence of spinal and spinal cord injuries and their surgical treatment in children and adolescents: a population-based study. *Spine (Phila Pa 1976).*, 2010, 35(1), 104-7.

[58] Uzun, N; Tanriverdi, T; Savrun, FK; Kiziltan, ME; Sahin, R; Hanimoglu, H; Hanci, M. Traumatic peripheral nerve injuries: demographic and electrophysiologic findings of 802 patients from a developing country. *J Clin Neuromuscul Dis.*, 2006, 7(3), 97-103.

[59] Kenny, SE; Tam, PK; Garcia-Barcelo, M. Hirschsprung's disease. *Semin Pediatr Surg.*, 2010, 19(3), 194-200.

[60] Kao, TCC; Chang, LW. The mechanism of spinal cord cavitation following spinal cord transection. *J Neurosurg.*, 1977, 46(2), 197-209.

[61] Shaw, D; Shoichet, MS. Toward spinal cord injury repair strategies: peptide surface modification of expanded poly(tetrafluoroethylene) fibers for guided neurite outgrowth in vitro. *J Craniofac Surg.*, 2003, 14(3), 308-16.

[62] Scholz, T; Krichevsky, A; Sumarto, A; Jaffurs, D; Wirth, GA; Paydar, K; Evans, GR. Peripheral nerve injuries: an international survey of current treatments and future perspectives. *J Reconstr Microsurg.*, 2009, 25(6), 339-44.

[63] Li, Q; Ping, P; Jiang, H; Liu, K. Nerve conduit filled with GDNF gene-modified Schwann cells enhances regeneration of the peripheral nerve. *Microsurgery.*, 2006, 26(2), 116-21.

[64] Radtke, C; Aizer, AA; Agulian, SK; Lankford, KL; Vogt, PM; Kocsis, JD. Transplantation of olfactory ensheathing cells enhances peripheral nerve regeneration after microsurgical nerve repair. *Brain Res.*, 2009, 1254, 10-7.

[65] Shi, Y; Zhou, L; Tian, J; Wang, Y. Transplantation of neural stem cells overexpressing glia-derived neurotrophic factor promotes facial nerve regeneration. *Acta Otolaryngol.*, 2008, 1-9.

[66] Keilhoff, G; Goihl, A; Langnäse, K; Fansa, H; Wolf, G. Transdifferentiation of mesenchymal stem cells into Schwann cell-like myelinating cells. *Eur J Cell Biol.*, 2006, 85(1), 11-24.

[67] Lankford, KL; Imaizumi, T; Honmou, O; Kocsis, JD. A quantitative morphometric analysis of rat spinal cord remyelination following transplantation of allogenic Schwann cells. *J Comp Neurol.*, 2002, 443(3), 259-74.

[68] Madduri, S; Gander, B. Schwann cell delivery of neurotrophic factors for peripheral nerve regeneration. *J Peripher Nerv Syst.*, 2010, 15(2), 93-103.

[69] Goto, E; Mukozawa, M; Mori, H; Hara, M. A rolled sheet of collagen gel with cultured Schwann cells: model of nerve conduit to enhance neurite growth. *J Biosci Bioeng.*, 2010, 109(5), 512-8.

[70] Huang, JH; Cullen, DK; Browne, KD; Groff, R; Zhang, J; Pfister, BJ; Zager, EL; Smith, DH. Long-term survival and integration of transplanted engineered nervous tissue constructs promotes peripheral nerve regeneration. *Tissue Eng Part A.*, 2009, 15(7), 1677-85.

[71] Iwata, A; Browne, KD; Pfister, BJ; Gruner, JA; Smith, DH. Long-term survival and outgrowth of mechanically engineered nervous tissue constructs implanted into spinal cord lesions. *Tissue Eng.*, 2006, 12(1), 101-10.

[72] Jandial, R; Snyder, EY. A safer stem cell: on guard against cancer. *Nat Med.*, 2009, 15(9), 999-1001.

[73] Alper, J. Geron gets green light for human trial of ES cell-derived product. *Nat Biotechnol.*, 2009, 27(3), 213-4.

[74] Zhang, YW; Denham, J; Thies, RS. Oligodendrocyte progenitor cells derived from human embryonic stem cells express neurotrophic factors. *Stem Cells Dev.*, 2006, 15(6), 943-52.

Editor's Contact Information

Dr. Sukhotnik Igor, M.D.
The Bruce Rappaport Faculty of Medicine
Technion-Israel Institute of Technology
Laboratory of Intestinal Adaptation and Recovery
Department of Pediatric Surgery
Bnai Zion Medical Center
47 Golomb St., P.O.B. 4940
Haifa, 31048, Israel
Tel: 972-4-8359647
Fax: 972-4-8359620
igor-dr@internet-zahav.net

Index

B

D

E

H

I

J

K

L

N

O

S

T

U

V